The Meditation Room

The Meditation Room

Enter Into Stillness and Discover the Peace Within

Jessica Bowles

Dedication

To all the teachers who experienced and shared the practice of yoga, helping to reveal and shape my understanding so I could implement the practice in my life and continue the tradition of sharing this gift with others. Special thanks to those who influenced me most—Erich Schiffman, for the foundational understanding of the purpose and application of the practice, and Michael Stone, for unveiling the depth and vividness of the practice.

And my deepest gratitude to my husband and children for all of their everflowing love and support of my growth, vision, and journey.

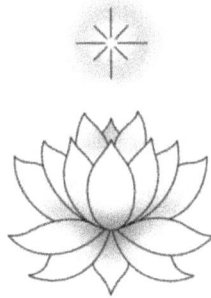

Contents

Introduction

The purpose of this book is to help you understand how to utilize the practice of meditation to create a peaceful baseline from which to live your life. While the science of yoga originated in ancient times and has its roots in India, its teachings are universal and still valid for us in modern day. The world around us has changed, yet we are still the same living beings—learning, loving, suffering, healing, and connecting—as we were thousands of years ago. Through the integrated system of yoga, we can discover how to live well and balanced in body, mind, and soul despite our everchanging circumstances. As we take in information from the world around us, our minds like to label and associate to past experience to make sense of the details. Yet this way of processing does not allow us to perceive new information with clarity. For this, we must widen our view of what we know and clear our perceptual lens. As you turn the pages of this book and absorb the information it entails, allow yourself to release any thoughts or past perceptions of meditation in order to experience every step with clear, fresh eyes.

Meditation is simply allowing your focus to rest on one object of attention, and there are many different ways to do this. Although, just like any other form of nourishment, it only helps if you do it! So, finding a practice that works for you is key. The practice of meditation shared within this book is derived from the yoga tradition with primary focus on teachings from *The Yoga Sutras of Patanjali*, the principles of *Raja Yoga* and its eight limbs of practice, and the study of the *koshas*. My goal is to offer these teachings in an accessible, tangible way to enable you to deeply nourish yourself and feel more balanced, peaceful, and at ease in your life. Through these concepts and practices, you can establish a daily routine of nurturing your whole being—body, mind, and soul.

The philosophy, concepts, and practices being offered are derived from the yoga tradition. While, in the West, yoga tends to be thought of as mainly a physical practice, the word *yoga* simply translates as "to unite, to yoke, to come together."[1] The physical practice of yoga, uniting movements with breath and mind with body awareness, is just one limb of the eight limbs of yoga practice. And while the yoga body postures are very important, instead of being a description of what yoga is, their main purpose is to help prepare the body to *not* be an obstacle to the mind in meditation or in life. Erich Schiffmann describes it best in his book *Yoga: The Spirit and Practice of Moving Into Stillness*: "When yoga was first being developed, the primary practice was meditation, or centering. The poses had not yet been invented. It was out of that centered awareness that the poses evolved. The ancient yogis were simply moved to do them as a result of their meditative practice. Then they practiced and taught these to others as a way of finding or returning to that centered meditative state. The asanas were not only valued because they were physically beneficial but because they were an especially effective way of both facilitating and sustaining the meditative states. The primary practice, however, was and is meditation...experiencing oneself in stillness."[2]

The philosophy and practices of yoga were first passed down from teacher to student until, around 400 CE, being recorded in sacred texts written in Sanskrit, an ancient language of India used for spiritual texts, such as the *Yoga Sutras of Patanjali* (which will be our primary focus here). Raja Yoga, the path of mind and meditation, is where we find the practices shared in this book. On this path, we utilize the steps and disciplines of the eight limbs of yoga, compiled by Sage Patanjali Maharishi in the *Yoga Sutras*. Each limb of yoga practice helps us move into a meditative state with more ease by strengthening our focus in order to not be so pushed and pulled by all of the external and internal elements of living that distract the mind. In this process, we also learn to release tensions in the body, old patterns of energetic holding, and mental clutter. As we continue to practice and experience the techniques, we refine our ability to be present and mindful throughout all aspects of life. The clarity we gain through practice helps us to experience life with a clear view. Through this, you are able to live authentically by understanding who you truly are, what your purpose is in this life, and how to move away from the need of external reassurance.

While each of the limbs can be practiced on their own, they work best as a progressive system. The first two practices involve your connection with the world around you and your connection with yourself. These help build a strong foundation for living and for successful outcomes using the techniques that follow. The third limb consists of practices that instill ease and stability in the physical body, the fourth practice supports the free flow of the energetic body, and the fifth practice develops an understanding of how to withdraw the senses from environmental distractions. The sixth involves creating an easeful focus of mind, and the final two practices occur as a byproduct of that previous one's success. They are the goal, the direction, and the outcome of all preceding practices. When we are able to move beyond the mental distractions of the body, energetic holdings, and environmental, sensory distractions to harness a continuous stream of mental focus, we reach the seventh limb of practice—meditative state. It is there that you will be able to connect to the deepest aspect of yourself, beneath worldly concerns and thoughts, and experience the eighth limb of practice—oneness with all, a deep feeling of non-separation, complete union, and the true meaning of *yoga*.

Welcome to The Meditation Room
Om Peace,
Jessica

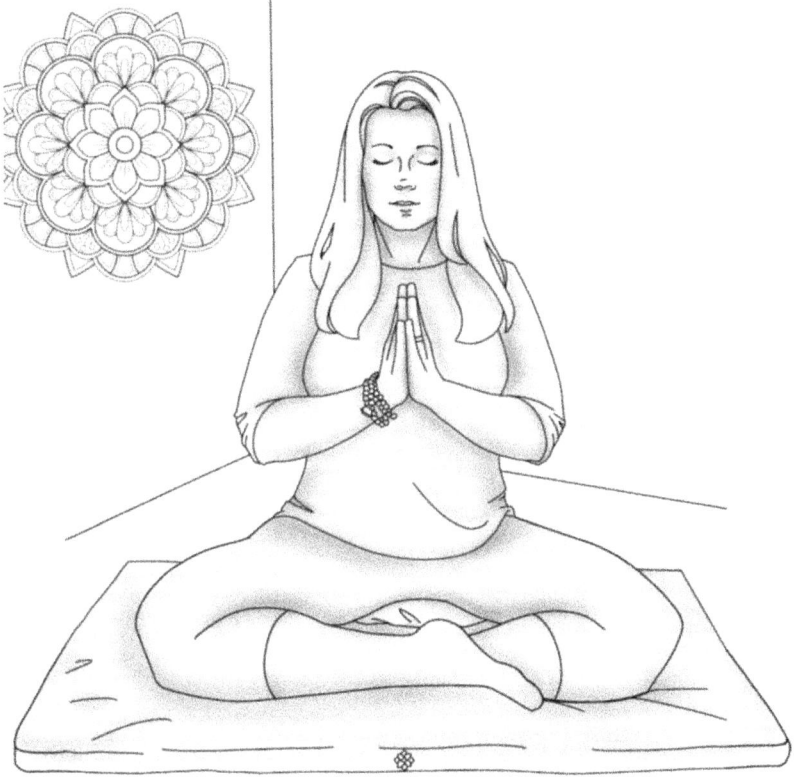

Chapter 1

Begin Where You Are

Take a few moments to connect with your surroundings.
With a soft, lowered gaze or eyes closed, notice the feeling of your environment—
ground beneath you, temperature of the air against your skin, any subtle sounds.

Observe the current feeling of your body...
soften and release any tension or holding you find.

Relax your jaw. Soften your eyes and forehead.
Notice the current state of the space behind eyes and forehead.
Observe the feeling of the space of your mind and begin to soften and release any tension or holding you find there as well.

Then begin to allow your focus to rest on the current feeling of your body effortlessly expanding and releasing with each natural breath.

The practice of meditation nourishes you wherever you are in your life and whatever state you are in. With a piece of fresh fruit, you do not need to be in a healthy, balanced state to benefit from its nutrients; you just need to eat it. With every bite, your body is a little more nourished. The more you add the fruit to your life, the more you receive its benefits. Meditation is helpful in this same way. Whatever your starting point is, if you utilize the practices, you will begin to move toward a healthy and balanced state. The key is to meet yourself where you are and practice. Whether it is your first time meditating or your millionth, awareness of your current state of being is crucial. From the first moment of meditation, as you close your eyes, you will notice *how your body feels*. You may observe tension in areas you have not even realized you are holding. Once you start reflecting inward and paying attention to your body, it will reveal to you any layers of unconscious holding, imbalance, or unease. You may notice sensations like tightness of breath, mental grasping at sounds in your environment, or the distraction of thoughts running through your mind. Note that these conditions have not occurred *because* you noticed them. They already existed, undetected under the noise of everyday distractions and mental chatter. If you do not listen to your body and mind, these imbalances only grow louder, so this ability to connect inward is truly a gift! To have insight into these subtle physical tensions and unease in the body before they become larger issues will help you keep your body more balanced and well.

Just as we all have the ability to connect to our outward environment through the five senses and take in information about the world around us, we also have another skill of sensing (a faculty through which the body perceives)—the ability to tune inward. Every one of us has this capability even if we are not yet aware of its depth. You are the only one who can perceive yourself in this way; therefore, it is incredibly important to connect inward to all aspects of yourself. The totality of how you feel and experience your daily life is an accumulation of all of the layers of yourself. These all must be nourished and balanced to cultivate a healthy baseline for living. Meditating strengthens this ability to tune in to your body, breath, thoughts, and mind space by directing your awareness inward.

Releasing Our Grasp

Through living, we encounter physical, mental, and emotional stressors that can create holding in breath patterns, physical tension, and mental grasping. This can occur even more drastically through living a life that is fast-paced and full of multitasking or constant environmental distractions. This is a common experience in modern-day life, as we tend to get into a habit of mentally operating in multitasker mode. We are thinking about something while driving, while eating, while talking, while listening, and so on. Yet the mind is a singular processor of information that can only focus on one thing at a time—it is just incredibly fast! While you may appear able to focus on many tasks at once, your *one-pointed* mind is just quickly bouncing around to all of the different points of your focus. This way of mentally operating is exhausting and prevents you from being fully present for any one of the many things your mind is trying to focus on. We are also creatures of habit, so if you are mentally functioning in this way for too long, your mind gets into deep grooves of processing in this way and it becomes difficult to focus, be mindful, and relax. *This is where the tool of meditation comes in.*

Through meditation, we are training the mind to be more focused and undistracted. As we continue to practice, this comes with more ease. The practice also helps to nourish and cleanse the mind of the daily clutter we gather through living. Our minds take in information all day long, from sights, sounds, tastes, and smells to experiences, emotions, and thoughts about those experiences and emotions. When looking at the mind as a functional processor of information, it is working hard around the clock. Consider a situation where you have to be on your feet all day—by the end of the day, your feet are in great need of rest. Similarly, your mind needs time to rest. Through the process of meditation, you allow your mind to take a break from the informational processing it does all day long and become better able to digest your daily experiences and emotions.

In the process of meditating, you are also creating a new mental habit—one that nourishes the mind, allows it to rest, and helps you be more focused, mindful, and present all of the rest of the time. Regardless of the type of technique you utilize, the practice of meditating is bringing your *one-pointed focus* to an object of attention and guiding it back whenever you notice distraction occurring. Through this, you begin to reach a meditative state. This can feel difficult, especially if it is not something your mind is accustomed to, yet—through practice— you will start to strengthen your ability to focus, not just in your practice but also in your life.

It is helpful to understand that we are continuously cultivating habits, whether we are trying to create them or not. In fact, how your mind is currently functioning has less to do with your cognitive ability and more with your current habits. Whatever mode of functioning your mind is in at this very moment is due to the mix of current habits you have cultivated. Modern life encourages us to live in multitasking mode. Once we develop this habit, it is difficult not to operate this way. Though it may seem, at times, that we can accomplish more while doing this, we are not truly present with any one of the many things we are quickly trying to focus on and it can be difficult to let go of this habit. When we want to focus, be present, relax, and release this mode of "doing," it can feel almost impossible to tap out of this scattered state. In these moments, it is important to realize this is not how your mind inherently works but just the current mental habit you have cultivated. Just as you can develop the habit of constantly shifting your focus, you can also create a habit of using a more present, controlled way of mental processing in your life.

Since we are forming mental habits all of the time, we have the ability to create new nourishing habits versus habits that deplete us. This may feel easier said than done, especially when it comes to subtle habits that have settled into well-worn grooves in the mind. Yet this is where our practice becomes pivotal, helping us to calm the distractions of the mind and discover the sources of their deep pull. This is not done through a process of searching and analyzing but rather through learning how to *ungrasp* (a term for releasing mental or physical clinging) what arises and eliminate old habits as we bring in new nurturing habits to fill their place.

One of the main habits that modern-day society tends to create and cultivate in our life is *tension.* We are prone to holding unnecessary tensions in the physical body and mind, which begin to intertwine and influence each other—when tension arises in the body, it directly affects the mind, and when there is holding in the mind, it will inevitably affect the body. We tend to be more aware of this deep connection through its negative effects. If you are experiencing intense pain in the body, your mind will go directly to the pain and it will be very difficult to focus on anything else. This physical pain can then begin to affect your mind, as you may become anxious, worried, or depressed. The same is also true if you are experiencing issues in your life causing feelings of stress in your mind. Your body will eventually begin to feel this stress in various forms, such as headaches, pain, and even illness. Yet once you become aware of this connection, you can use it to your benefit. You can learn to release your physical and mental holdings through the concept of ungrasping. Just like the ability to let go of an object held tight in your hand, you also have this ability to release the tension or thoughts you are grasping on to in the mind.

This idea of ungrasping in mind and body forms the basis for the practice of non-attachment. This practice is the process in which we release our grip on old ideas, viewpoints, dialogue, patterns, and habits. It is also what gives us the ability to notice the grasping of mind and body in the first place. Witnessing our patterns of attachment and holding in our physical, energetic, and mental bodies is the first step to dissolving them.

If you are not aware of the holding and clinging occurring within yourself, you will only notice the negative outcomes they produce, such as stress, habitual thought patterns and reactions, and even pain due to the mind being stuck in the cycle of grasping itself. It is in the quiet moments of practice, when we are able to witness the feeling of body, our natural breath, and our space of mind, that we discover where we are unconsciously holding and mentally grasping. This is when we strengthen our ability to ungrasp at any given moment, both inside and outside of practice, forming more beneficial habits and patterns for clarity and focus throughout life.

This process starts by directing our awareness inward and simply noticing. This first step is, at times, the biggest leap to practice. The reason why many of us stay in a mode of distraction and do not take the time to connect inwardly is a bit purposeful—to avoid becoming any more aware of discomfort in body or chaos in mind. However, just like when we procrastinate cleaning up dirty dishes or taking out the trash, the issue doesn't go away; it just builds up, becomes harder to clean, and may start to creep into other areas of the house. Once we are able to notice any unconscious holding or imbalance is when we can release it and the process of unraveling the tensions of body and mind begins. When the body softens, the mind begins to relax and release whatever thoughts or dialogue it is holding on to as well. If you are able to ungrasp the thoughts in your mind, then you will start to release the physical tension in your body. The connection between mind and body is strong. Learn to utilize this reality for more positive outcomes in your life by nourishing and balancing both aspects of yourself. By increasing your awareness of the mind-body connection, you will notice grasping with more ease and become more adept at softening it when it begins to arise.

The main area of the body where we find a direct connection to mind is the mouth. In his teachings, Michael Stone describes how to use the method of ungrasping in mind and throughout the body by revealing, "We begin to mentally ungrasp with the small adjustments in the tongue, the soft palate, and the way muscles hold the bones. These physical adjustments in form and attitude start to *make space in the mind*."[1] When there is grasping in the mind, tension will occur in the body—first in the mouth, second in the hands, and then throughout the body. The mouth reflects any tension in mind, the hands reflect the mouth, and so on. To look a little deeper into this concept, there is an even more specific area of the body considered the "physical seat of the mind."[2] This is the roof of the mouth, or soft palate, which directly reflects the current state of mind. By tapping into this tell of the body, you can attune to the state of your mind at any time and release whatever you are holding on to. For example, if you become angry or worried, grasping on to these emotional thoughts will cause tension to arise in your soft palate, then in your jaw and tongue, and eventually in your hands. In the opposite case, when witnessing something beautiful like a sunset or someone you love, your mind begins to open and a feeling of awe causes the soft palate to naturally lift and widen. This amazing technique can be utilized at any time. If you feel that tension is developing in your mind or you find yourself continuously distracted in your meditation practice, soften hands, relax your whole mouth, and feel the roof of your mouth lift and widen.

Creating Space

As you cultivate more space and ease within, this starts to ripple out into other aspects of yourself. When you feel more open and spacious in your body and mind, you feel more healthy and balanced. Yet if you are tight in your muscles and joints and cannot move as freely as you should, you begin to hurt and do not function as well. In your energetic (subtle) body, creating space enables your life force to flow through you with ease so you feel good, open, and balanced. You can use this same concept for creating a more spacious mind. Unhealthy mental states, such as anger, depression, or frustration, feel very constricting and confining. On the other hand, healthy mental states, such as calmness, love, and joy, feel open, expansive, and spacious. The process of learning how to mentally ungrasp in your meditation practice helps you allow your mind to remain calm and spacious through all other moments in your life. As your practice develops, you will begin to tap into this feeling and awareness with more ease.

Effortless Posture

Your practice will help you with not only creating a more spacious sense of being but also with connecting to your current state to meet yourself where you are and gradually release your grasp, allowing the expansion to occur. Your physical body is of utmost importance, as it marks the first step that begins the flow of release and is also your foundation for continuing the inward journey. For your meditation practice, find a comfortable upright position in an effortless seated posture. Laying down for a meditation is lovely; it just offers a different benefit. When we are in a supine position, our energy begins to spread out and we are able to relax deeply, so much so that we may dip down into an unconscious or sleep state. While laying down for practice is a helpful way to rest and relax into sleep with more ease, we are moving toward a slightly different outcome. We sit in our practice because this is how we live our lives, upright and conscious. When your spine is upright, your energy is flowing up and down, opening and expanding. In this way, you are conscious and moving toward strengthening your focus and clearing the clutter of attachments and distractions.

Everything that you are learning and experiencing in your practice aims to help you feel this way all of the time, so developing a practice that supports the way you are in your daily life is key. In a comfortable seated posture, you are able to tap into how you hold your body and consciously create more space by loosening your grip on unnecessary tension you may find. Once you cultivate this stability and ease in the body through your practice, you will gradually begin to hold your body in this way all of the time. As you discover how to relax your daily tensions, you will start to create a state of being that does not collect all of this tension in the first place. If tension does accumulate, you can release it with more ease because you are witnessing it from a more balanced state.

We approach this very differently than most things we are trying to achieve. For most of our lives, we must *do* in order to accomplish a task, yet when it comes to meditation practice, it is a process of *not doing* that allows us to find a "perfect posture." The best approach is to notice the unnecessary doing of the body and begin a process of *not doing* it any more. Oftentimes, we bring unnecessary tension into our bodies that is not needed. Ingrid Bacci wonderfully reveals this concept in her book *The Art of Effortless Living* as she guides you through a simple exercise to experience the feeling of effortless stability in your hand. After having you write your name with pen and paper, she leads you through completely relaxing your hand while still holding your pen. She then asks you to keep your hand in this totally relaxed state and, once again, write your name. Through this experience, you will realize that you can, in fact, still sign your name (and possibly even better) without all of the effort and tension you were putting into it. We do many things with our bodies in this same manner—from activities to simply sitting in a chair, we often add too much unnecessary "doing" in our physical bodies that is not helpful or required.

Our goal in practice is to find a state of physical being that is *effortless*. You start by finding a comfortable way to support your body in seated posture. It is important to find support for your current state, meaning what your body needs to be able to sit in an effortless way. For example, when you meet your body where it is by adding support under the knees so the hips can relax or support for the back so you can be upright with more ease, this allows your hips to release or your back to strengthen. Eventually, your body may no longer need these supports. In other cases, you may begin your practice not needing any added support but then find them necessary after an injury or another physical change. Meet yourself where you are. Specific seated postures are further described in Chapter 2.

Once you find a comfortable seat and begin to notice unnecessary holding and tension in your body, there are two gentle techniques that can help to start the gradual loosening of effort and allow your body to settle. The first takes place simply through your awareness. Just noticing the holding and bringing your attention to it gives you the ability to release. It is your *un*awareness that allows it to collect and stay there; it is your awareness that allows you to let it go. As your body softens, your grasp on the things around you will become apparent. Until you close your eyes and begin to tune inward, your awareness is focused on the world around you. The next step is loosening your grip of anything around you that your mind may be holding on to. To do this, gently expand your awareness of all things by mentally stepping back and spreading your awareness outward. Instead of placing your awareness on one thing, allow it to gently observe all that is without grasping or landing on anything. This is not something that you will necessarily accomplish, due to your one-pointed processor mind, yet trying to do it will create a releasing effect that helps you sink deeper into an effortless state.

Be Easy on Yourself

This is a practice of undoing old habits, loosening the knots, releasing unconscious holds, and clearing out old energetic and mental clutter. Be easy on yourself. It has taken you a while to arrive at the current state you are in, and it will take time to gradually discover and discard the habits and clutter you find. *Be easy on yourself.* It is not about the destination; the journey is what is of most importance, for the destination you are moving toward is always *now*. Life is continuously flowing, so you are always simultaneously on the journey and at your destination. The best way to begin to infuse these practices into your life is to create space for them. Set aside a time each day, yet also be flexible with yourself. There are benefits to having a regularly scheduled routine—finding a specific time each day to set aside for practice will help you adjust to a new habit. Yet also be gentle with yourself and ease it into your day naturally. When this is not possible, allow for flexibility and whatever works for that day's schedule. It is also helpful to keep your cushion in a special space or room that you go to every day while allowing it to travel between different spots in your home, areas outdoors, or possibly a local meditation center that offers open times for personal practice.

Chapter 2

The Practice

At this moment, notice how your body feels.
Is there anywhere in your body that is tense or
unnecessarily holding?
Soften there and begin to allow your physical body to
settle and relax.
Notice how you can continue to be upright, steady in
body, yet also be soft and at ease.

As you continue to read these words…
allow your lips to part, just a little bit, to release your jaw.
Relax your tongue and feel the whole mouth soften.
Begin to release any holding in the eyes and forehead.

Now begin to observe your body breathing. Without trying to
change the breath, just notice it naturally moving in and out of the
body. Observe the steady calm of this effortless movement.

We tend to think of ourselves and others as the tangible bodies we feel, see, and experience life through, yet the physical body does not create a living human experience. We are also energetic systems of automatic functioning and consciousness that, together with our physical bodies, create human life. Each of these aspects of us cannot exist without the others or thrive without the nourishment of all. With the practices of the eight limbs of yoga, we can nurture each level of our being individually and as part of a whole system. The goal of this practice is to move into a state of meditation with more ease by gradually learning how to ungrasp from all of the distractions typically tugging at the mind.

We live in a world of information and technology always at our fingertips with our focus being continuously pushed and pulled by the outside world in addition to feelings in our bodies, emotions, and inner dialogue. With all of this distraction, the mind can feel crowded and, at times, chaotic, which makes it incredibly difficult to see, experience, and find peace in our lives. In the *Yoga Sutras of Patanjali*, the space of mind is described as a calm and tranquil pond, and every time the mind is distracted, it creates a ripple in the water. If the water is wavy and chaotic, it is difficult to be present and focused. In this state of mind, not only is your perception of life clouded, but it is also difficult to connect within to who you truly are. You begin to think that *you are* the ripples and waves (thoughts and emotions) you feel in mind space. Meditation helps you to *calm the fluctuations of the mind so your perception becomes clear*. With nothing clouding your view, you can then experience life with clarity as well as experience your *true self,* free from all of the thoughts and emotions swirling around in mind space. The practice helps you calm the waters of the mind through cultivating focus so that the ripples are less.

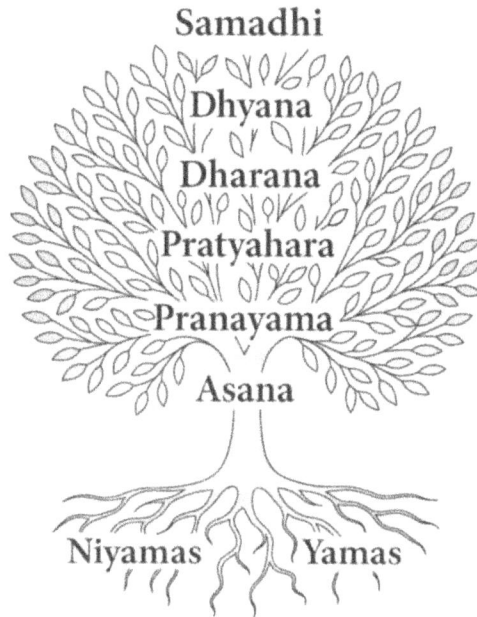

Samadhi
Dhyana
Dharana
Pratyahara
Pranayama
Asana
Niyamas   Yamas

The Eight Limbs of Yoga

The path of Raja Yoga is a systematic method to finding health, balance, and union in your whole being with an emphasis on meditation and gaining access to your true self (free from physical distractions, emotions, and thoughts). To strengthen your ability to meditate and reach what lies beneath distraction and the ripples of mind space, there are eight specific tools to use along the way. These eight techniques are described both as "rungs," used sequentially as when climbing a ladder, and "limbs" that, like the branches of a tree, can grow simultaneously or individually. These aspects of utilizing the techniques are important for gaining foundational benefits and longevity of the practice.

To begin to move inward to a calm and peaceful state of mind, there are layers of distraction we must move through. These levels of our being that the mind encounters are found in a very specific order. Just like the layers of an onion, one must be peeled back or surpassed before accessing the next. Luckily, our tools and techniques in the eight limbs of yoga help us along the way, each guiding us through a specific layer of distraction with more ease in order to reach the next.

The first aspect that you will encounter as you begin to turn your awareness inward is your physical body. Beyond just noticing the feelings of the body, if you are not able to release its pull of awareness, create softness, and peel back the layer of distraction of the physical body, then you will not be able to access any of your deeper aspects…your awareness will remain focused on how the body feels. And if you are not able to access deeper layers, even in your meditation practice, the body is where you will feel that your Self starts and ends. Therefore, you will experience life through the mindset that you are this body and everything relating to and affecting the physical self. Yet this is only the first layer, the first step to understanding and experiencing the depth of what you truly are and can access within. To be able to move beyond simple body awareness and develop a more expansive view of yourself and your depth, there is a specific yogic technique known as *asana,* defined as "posture; to sit; to become established in a particular position."[1] This limb of practice offers postures for the body to help you move through this first layer, keeping it healthy and open.

Yoga Asana

While yoga asana is often thought of as one of two extremes— either intense active practice or simply stretching—the actual goal of the technique is to create a state of body that is *not an obstacle to the mind in meditation.* There are many different aspects of our bodies that can cause pain, discomfort, and distraction, so the scope of postures is wide, as they can be utilized to strengthen our muscles, stretch and open the connective tissue (fascia) that makes us feel tight, and aid in deep relaxation and release. The element that forms the foundation of all of these aspects is cultivating a state of physical body that is not a distraction for the mind.

By practicing yoga asana, we get better at being able to release the tugs of bodily distractions during meditation as well as all of the rest of the time. The stability and ease that you are able to find in your body during practice will stay with you for a time. Then you will begin to create a new "normal" for how you hold your body and how your body supports you. When you experience how to consciously bring more steadiness and comfort to your body during practice, you can begin to cultivate that same state whenever you feel unbalanced and tense. It is a process of bringing your physical body to a more balanced *baseline of feeling* so that, as you move through the ever-changing elements of life, you will be able to process your experiences from a more stable and easeful state. By continuing the practice, you will find yourself staying close to that baseline.

By approaching the practice of asana at its foundation, you are able to utilize gentle, accessible postures for any current state your body is in with the purpose of finding a comfortable seat for meditation. The main measure of the quality of your posture, the way you hold your body while in a yoga asana, is that you feel physically steady and comfortable. This feeling of stability and ease is what we are aiming to create in the body with every pose. Through this, the tugs of physical distraction become less. When the body relaxes, the mind begins to soften as well. We are then able to start the process of releasing the grasp of both. There are subtle distinctions between the bodily approach you use in yoga asana and other styles of movements or postures. You accept yourself where you are in each moment, discover your ever-changing starting point, and adjust the pose to your body (never the reverse). In this way, the practice is accessible to any *body* and any support that body requires. The postures are also practiced progressively, starting where you are and guiding you into a more stable and comfortable state.

Another main component of the practice is uniting your postures and the movement in and out of each with your breath. In his book *The Heart of Yoga*, renowned yoga teacher T. K. V. Desikachar states, "The breath is the link between the inner and outer body. It is only by bringing body, breath, and mind into unison that we realize the true quality of an asana."[2] When you join your active breath with each asana and link your focus to this union, it enhances your ability to soften and release. You begin this by simply bringing your awareness to the feeling of natural breath, gradually deepening each inhale and lengthening each following exhale, and allowing the postures to bloom out of that rhythm and awareness. When practiced in this way, there is no need to count or keep a pace, as every movement and pause is led by the breath. As you allow your body to breathe at its full capacity, with each inhale filling the lungs completely and each exhale releasing every last drop of breath, you are also releasing unconscious physical holdings that may have accumulated through short, shallow breathing. Linked to breath and body, the mind now has a place to focus and settle as its wandering habit begins to subside.

We utilize asana in two main ways. The practice includes many different movement postures to achieve a release of body and specific asanas for our seated meditation practice. The active asana helps us to find an asana for seated practice with more comfort and ease. There are a variety of options to support your body in seated practice. The key components are that you feel stable in your base (hips and legs), that your spine feels long and upright, and that you can be at ease in your body (with no need of holding or doing). It is helpful to support and level your hips with a cushion, bench, or chair. If you are on a cushion and your knees can be bent, make sure to allow one foot to rest in front of the other (not crossed) with your knees supported, if not on the floor. If you need to straighten your legs, lean against a wall or use a floor chair. These two options are also helpful if you need extra back support. Sitting in a regular chair is another option if coming down to the floor is not available to you due to your body or space. If you are in a chair, make sure that your feet feel level with the ground and supported; if not, place something under them. It is helpful to first find this comfortable seat for meditation before utilizing postures to gently release all directions of the spine with active breath so that you can return to it with ease and sink into your stillness.

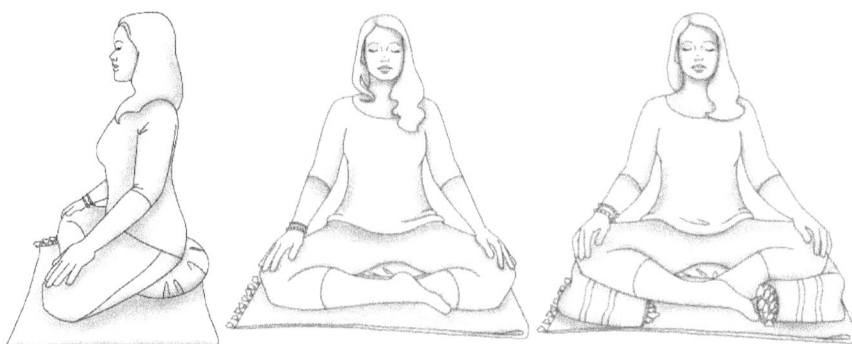

Easy Pose
(*Sukhasana*) *Sukha* translated as "easy" and *asana* meaning "posture." Sitting on a meditation cushion is helpful to support the hips and create length in the spine.

With knees bent, bring one foot in front of the other (legs not crossed) and allow the hands to rest palms down on the knees. A blanket or soft surface under the legs is also helpful.

If your knees do not touch the floor, placing support under them (such as folded blankets) can alleviate stress on the hips. If you need to straighten your legs and/or need more back support, lean against a wall.

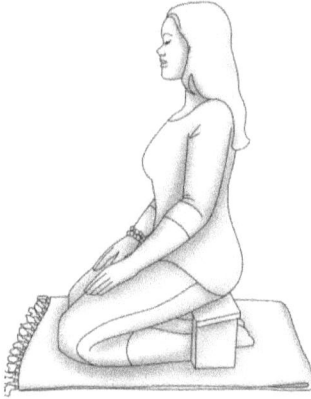

Hero Pose (*Virasana*) *Vira* is defined as "brave" and *asana* as "pose." This posture can also be utilized for meditation and is commonly used with a meditation bench for support under the hips to alleviate pressure in the knees and lower back. Contraindications are tightness or any injury to ankles or knees.

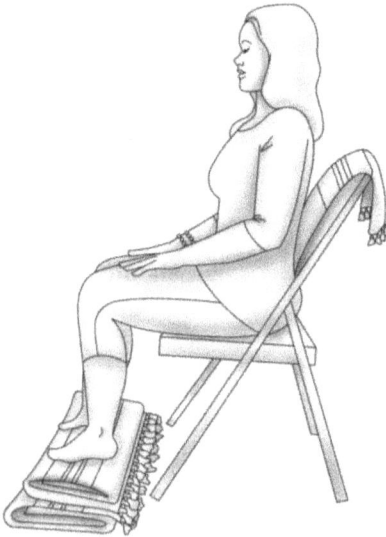

Sitting in a chair is also an option if coming down to the floor is not available to you due to your body or space.

Make sure your seat is a stable surface and your back is upright (not slouching). Place a folded blanket lengthwise to support the spine, if needed. Your feet should feel level with the ground and supported; if not, place something under them so that your knees are in line with your hips. Rest your hands on the thighs.

To release the distraction of physical holding and tension, you must go to the source—the spine, which is the true physical baseline of how you feel in your body. If there is holding or misalignment that prevents you from moving with ease in your spine, it will start to radiate pain or discomfort into the rest of the body. Likewise, if pain exists in other areas of the body, such as the shoulders, hips, or knees, it will eventually cause restrictions in the movements of the spine. To meet the body wherever it is and create a state of comfort from that point onward, you can utilize asana to bring gentle alignment and release to all six main movements of the spine: lateral, rotation to the right and left, and flexion forwards and backwards.

To expand from just trying to move in a direction and create a yoga asana that specifically releases holding and tension in the spine, we bring conscious alignment cues and breath awareness to each movement. We start by bringing awareness inward to the *feeling of body and feeling of breath:*

Close your eyes and allow your awareness to gradually move inward, observing the current feeling of your body. Anywhere you may find unnecessary holding or tension, start to consciously soften, consciously release.
Begin to feel the lower body (hips & legs) release and ground into the support beneath you while, at the same time, the top of the head gradually reaches up toward the sky.
Then allow your shoulders to drop away from the ears, creating a feeling of length in the neck and a softening of the chest.
Feel all the muscles of the face relax and release.

*Then begin to notice the feeling of your body effortlessly
breathing.
Observe the current rhythm of your belly, gentle expansion
and release of the ribs,
the subtle rise and fall of chest, even connecting to the
feeling of
natural breath gliding in and out of your nose.*

*Continuing to observe the feeling of breathing, on your next
inhale through the nose, begin to deepen the breath.
On the following exhale through the nose, start to lengthen
the breath. Continue to keep your awareness inward on this
deep, full breath as you move.*

The key aspect of moving in and out of asana, which helps us
continue to cultivate a state of stability and comfort, is joining the
breath to every posture and every transition, adding an inhale to
your movement any time you lengthen and rise, followed by an
exhale as you fold, bend, or twist. This breath awareness also
reminds us to lengthen the upper body before every movement to
keep the spine long, open, and safe.

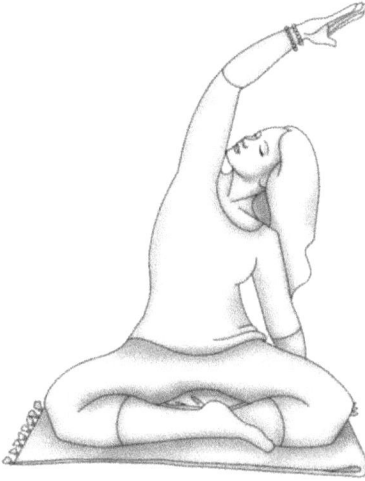

~ Laterals ~

On a big deep inhale, reach the right arm up and lengthen the right-side waist. Keep that length, and on your full, complete exhale, laterally bend to the left, leaning into your left hand, whether on the floor, chair, or the side of your leg.

Feel the right hip (or foot if standing) grounding into the floor. Allow for a gentle tilt of the chin toward the sky to open the chest.

On a deep, full inhale, rise, coming back to that length in the right-side waist. Keep that feeling of length, yet on your complete exhale, lower your arm down. Repeat on the left side.

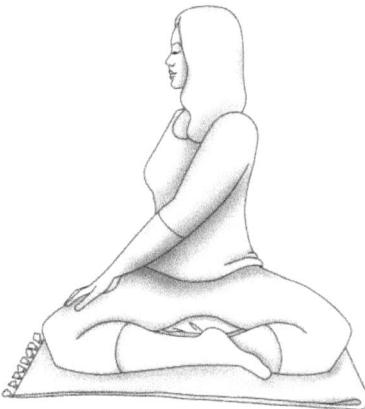

~ Twists ~

On a deep, full inhale, feel the top of the head lifting toward the sky to find length in the spine. Keep that length, yet on your full, complete exhale, allow your heart to face toward the right, your left hand coming to your right leg somewhere and your right hand coming behind you. Stay in this gentle twist for a breath.

Inhale…feeling the crown of your head moving toward the sky.

Exhale…feel the heart opening just a little more. Slowly unwind back to center and repeat on the left side.

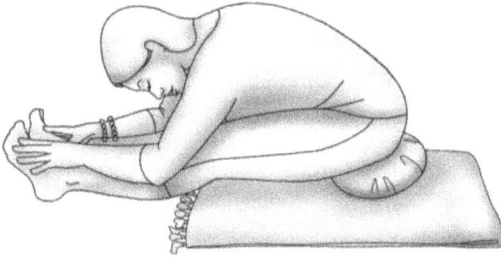

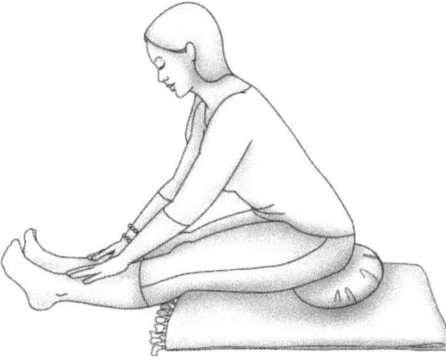

~ Flexion ~

Allowing your legs to be long, take a deep inhale to lengthen the spine. On your exhale, hinge forward from the hips. Once you go as far as your hips will allow, soften in your lower back, mid-back, upper back, release any tension in the back of your neck, and relax your face. Staying in the relaxed feeling of a forward fold, on your next full inhale, rise just enough to find length in your spine. On your following complete exhale, fully release your body back into the fold.

~ Seated Posture/Asana for Stillness ~

Gently return to your starting comfortable seated posture. Making sure hips feel level, knees are supported, and spine is long, release any movement of body and continue with your inward gaze, utilizing a specific active breathing technique.

Pranayama

Once you are able to release the distraction of the body, the next aspect of yourself that your mind will connect with is your *prana* layer. This is your "life force," the aspect of energy moving through you that makes you a living being, the same energy that is moving through and animating all life around us. It is the aspect of you that can feel depleted, blocked, low…or open, vibrant, and alive! This layer is the connection of body and mind that allows them to work together as a whole functioning, living being. Prana flows in and out of your body through your breath, yet it is also the power behind how your body naturally breathes. To connect to it, you bring your mind and awareness to the natural feeling of the body breathing. The current amount of prana flowing freely through you depends on how deeply and freely your body is breathing. Because of this, you have the ability to adjust and change the current level of prana within you through your breath.

A low quality of prana within is cultivated by incorrect breathing, not utilizing our lungs to their full capacity. When we are stressed, we begin to take more short, shallow breaths. While this type of breathing occurs as a response to stress, we can also get into a habit of breathing this way, which can then create a response in the mind and body causing feelings of anxiety, fatigue, or energetic tension and holding. Developing a habit of chest breathing tends to occur from living a stressful or fast-paced life. If this is the case, once you connect to this layer, it may feel like a brick wall is keeping you from moving any deeper into your practice. These feelings were already there, possibly even lying beneath the surface of your conscious awareness. Yet the current state of how you energetically feel reveals itself when you pay attention to it. Just as in the body, our busy lives are a distraction that causes us not to notice subtle imbalances in how we feel until they become loud. While connecting into our *unease* can feel uncomfortable, it is only by bringing our awareness to it that we can start to release it. Becoming aware of your current energetic state is the first step to instilling balance before there is a disturbance.

In your practice, once you connect to the energetic quality of *how you feel*, it can become such a distraction that moving beyond this and being able to meditate may feel impossible. After making the connection, the next step is doing something to create more balance. The specific technique of *pranayama* helps to create a calm pranic layer. This more open and balanced energetic state removes barriers and distractions in order to move deeper into your meditation practice. The practice of pranayama, or yogic breathing techniques, is a tool designed to adjust, shift, and change the quality of prana within. To be able to increase your pranic flow is incredibly helpful because whether its level is high or low determines how you feel in mind and body as well as how you operate. This is mostly due to your state of mind's direct link to the quality of prana within you. If your energy is low, your mind can feel restless, confused, unwell, stuck, and lacking in motivation. On the other hand, if you have more prana within, your mind feels peaceful, well-balanced, light, and vibrant! You may remember a time when you had a busy and stressful day and by the end of that day you felt spent, like your energetic cup was empty and you had nothing else to give—this is an immediate response to *low prana* within. Now think back to how amazing you felt after an aerobic exercise, breathwork, or yoga practice—this is the immediate feeling of *high prana* within.

We feel best when our prana energy is flowing freely throughout the whole body, in the movement of our muscles, function of our organs, balance in our nervous system, ease of our breath, and open clarity of our mind. Having the ability to influence this flow through our breath means that we have so much more control over how we "feel" than we may have ever realized. There is no more just "waiting until it passes" as if there is nothing you can do or thinking that this is just who you are. All of your yogic practices, especially your breathwork practices, are the precise tools that adjust, shift, or change how you *energetically feel* to a higher, more balanced level every day and whenever you need it. With the practice of pranayama techniques, you have the ability to stay in a balanced pranic state most of the time. Then, when you feel any sort of imbalance, you have the clarity needed to be able to recognize it more quickly as well as the tools to return to a high-quality, balanced state with more ease. If the baseline of feeling in which you are experiencing your life is in a good state, then you are better equipped to handle and release any negative energy or suffering that you encounter and be truly present in all of the joyous, happy, loving moments as well.

Cultivating a heightened state of prana within not only helps you create greater flow throughout the body and mind but also helps you rid yourself of whatever, energetically, may be blocking the path of flow. This allows an energetic clearing to take place, helping you let go of old energetic patterns or stories in body and mind that you have been knowingly (or unknowingly) holding on to, in order to release what you no longer need. This occurs throughout the whole body—every aspect of you—from opening your chakras (the main energy centers of the body) to clearing the clutter of thoughts that have been clouding the mind. This is so beneficial for healthy, balanced living and incredibly helpful in our eight-limb process of preparing the mind for deep meditation. We begin by learning the foundation of "correct" expansive breathing. For each of the following breathing techniques, begin by creating deep, full inhales and long complete exhales and then add different aspects to expand the benefits. Approaching the practice in this way will help you connect to your ability to create new, improved breathing patterns and experience the benefit of bringing more prana within, then releasing it all to allow for more space in the next breath.

All of the following breathing techniques are recommended for one to three minutes, gradually extending up to five minutes over time. Always listen to your body, go slow, and be mindful.

~ Three-Part Breath ~
A wonderful technique to help you experience the full capacity of your lungs, it starts by meeting yourself where you are and gradually expands your capacity. This is the counter of chest breathing and helps us reverse this habit.

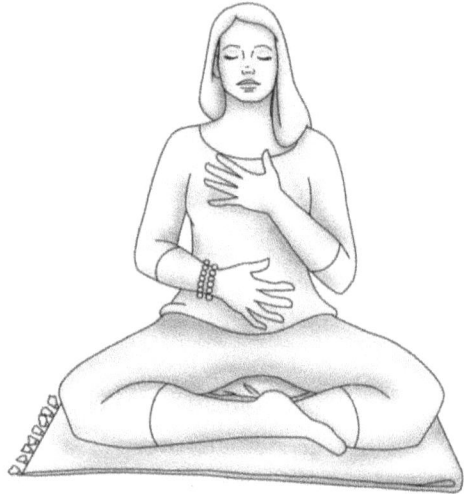

Imagine your lungs as a balloon. As you start blowing air into the balloon, it first expands at the bottom (belly), then the middle (ribs)...lastly the top (chest) until it is completely full. Then, as you release the air from the balloon, it deflates in reverse...chest, ribs, belly. Bring one hand to your belly, one hand to your heart, and begin to breathe in this way: On an inhale through the nose, expand in the belly, ribs, then the chest...
on your exhale through the nose release in the chest, ribs, belly. Continue these deep, full, expansive and complete breaths.

~ Suspension Breath ~
For this technique, you release awareness of the balloon and how you are breathing and simply begin with deepening your inhales and lengthening your exhales. Then you gradually add a subtle pause (hover) at the top of every inhale and another gentle pause (hover) at the bottom of every exhale. Make sure no tension arises

31

in your body with the pause. Rather, allow your body to soften with the suspension of breath.

Bring your awareness to the natural, effortless feeling of the body breathing, gradually lengthening each inhale through the nose and deepening each following exhale through the nose…gradually adding at the top of each inhale a subtle pause, then at the bottom of each exhale a subtle pause. Continuing with these four parts of your breath, inhale…pause….exhale….pause.

~ Ocean Breath ~

This breathing technique is known as *ujjayi* pranayama and translates as "victory breath."[3] It is helpful for creating mental focus, subtle internal heat, and balance. Start with your deep, full breath and then begin to add an ocean sound by creating a gentle constriction in the back of the throat (something that happens naturally when you fog up a mirror). Try this: Imagine you are trying to fog up a mirror with the breath coming out of your mouth. Now do this same thing but fog the mirror with the breath coming out of your nose. Continue with this gentle constriction in the throat as you exhale and inhale. The subtle ocean sound should be soft without creating any tension in your face or throat. It is especially helpful to utilize this during asana practice, as it allows you to keep your focus turned inward through the subtle sound even as you are moving.

Observe the current state of your natural breath.
Then start to gradually deepen each inhale and lengthen each exhale.
Continuing this full, complete breath, begin to add your ocean sound.
Make sure your body and face stay soft and relaxed even though your breath is active and full.

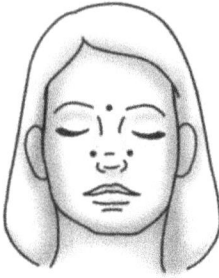

~ Alternate Nostril Breath ~
This breathing technique is also known as *nadi shodhana* pranayama. *Nadi* is a Sanskrit word meaning "passage" while *shodhana* means "cleansing."[4] It is a helpful way to clear and purify the subtle channels of your mind and body while also balancing the right (masculine/sun/yang) and the left (feminine/moon/yin) aspects of your energy. In this practice, you utilize your thumb and ring fingers to navigate your breath in and out of the nostrils by gently pressing the nadi points.

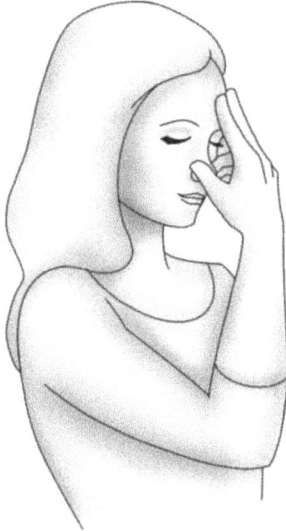

Bring your pointer finger and middle finger to your third-eye point at the center of the forehead, in between the eyebrows.
Closing off the right side, take a big deep inhale through the left...
close off the left, and exhale completely through the right...
inhale through the right, then close it off...
exhale through the left. This is a complete cycle.
Continue at your own pace,
allowing your last exhale to exit the same side as you began.

Pratyahara ~ Withdrawal of the Senses

Once you are able to release the distraction of your energetic body, the next thing you will notice is all of the sounds, textures, and smells in your environment through the pull of the senses. This next aspect that you will connect with is the *layer of your automatic mind (*the five senses). In this aspect of your mind, you do not have to consciously think to engage the senses; it happens automatically. This is a helpful way to expansively and effortlessly take in information from your environment. Similar to your body needing rest to maintain its strength, it is important for the mind to be able to release the tugs of your surroundings to strengthen your focus and connect deeper. If you are unable to release this pull of your attention, like an itchy sock, the smell of someone cooking, the sound of a ticking clock, the hum of a lawn mower, or a dog scratching at the door, it can be a barrier to your mind in meditation. To be in a space that is calm and quiet with very little outward distraction is helpful, but the goal is not only to be able to meditate when all of the conditions in your environment are perfectly void of distraction but also to learn how to be in the midst of chaos and still find peace.

Instead of removing yourself from distractions, you can learn how to ungrasp the pull of the senses with the next limb of yoga known as *pratyahara*. In this practice, you are creating the conditions for your senses to release their grip and to begin to withdraw inward. *Prati* is translated as "against or away" and *ahara* as "nourishment,"[5] so it is through this practice that you develop more control over what you take in from your environment through the senses. When you strengthen your ability to do this, you can cultivate a greater state of equanimity in your life by stepping out of reactivity and being so easily swayed by what is going on around you. This then allows you to move into a more balanced baseline of being for all of your experiences, whether wonderful or stressful. We get better at this in our

34

meditation practice so that we can also become less distracted by the world, living from a space of calm and peace.

Have you ever felt that it was too quiet or that silence was uncomfortable and you needed some distraction? Our senses are not only continually taking in information but are also forming habits through our patterns of interaction, creating the feeling that we *need* this stimulation of the senses from our environment. The practice of pratyahara helps us create a new habit where the senses no longer depend on these diversions and are not drawn away by them anymore. When we are able to release this connection, instead of our focus pinpointing and grasping on to specific distractions, it is as if we have mentally taken a step back and all of the distractions have become less attractive and easier to ignore so we are not as influenced. This limb of yoga practice prepares the mind for meditation by training it not to be attracted to environmental disturbances and helps us be less distracted and reactive in our daily lives.

From the moment you close your eyes and start to guide your awareness inward, the practice of pratyahara begins and all of the following limbs of the practice help cultivate this gradual withdrawal of the senses. You begin by guiding your focus to the feelings and movements of the body through asana. Then, once the mind is focused on the sensations of body and breath, the senses start to follow it. This also occurs in your pranayama practices, during which your focus is completely absorbed in the breath, creating an automatic release of the pull of outward attention. By the time you reach the step of practice where you cease all movement and active breathing, you have already begun to cultivate a state of being for pratyahara to occur. You are then able to become immersed in this state by utilizing specific techniques that continue to draw the senses inward toward your one-pointed focus. This step of practice helps your mind to rest and move into a meditative state with more ease and also helps you develop the ability to bring yourself back to that state if environmental distractions arise.

We each already have this ability, and we have all experienced it occurring naturally, such as when we are immersed in a movie, conversation, art project, or even a thought and may not hear someone call our name, see someone come into the room, or smell food cooking. Even if for a moment, our senses naturally disengage when the mind is completely focused on something. Yet, if this is not an ability you connect to often and if you do not allow this release from time to time, you may develop a habit of seeking constant engagement or even a state of feeling the need for sensory distraction. Through this limb of practice, there are many techniques and tools to help you connect to this ability and strengthen your capacity to release the tug of the senses by gaining greater control over what you take in from your environment.

We begin in our practice by closing our eyes. You do not have to close your eyes to meditate or experience withdrawal of the senses (there are specific practices where the eyes remain open), yet—since we take in so much information through our sight—it is helpful to close them, especially when you are beginning the practice. Once your eyes close, you begin to draw your focus inward by noticing the current feeling and sensations of the body. Then you begin to consciously release areas in the body related to mental tension by bringing your awareness to these areas and letting go of any unnecessary holding there. You start by softening and grounding into your foundation (the hips and legs), growing long through the spine, relaxing the shoulders, and releasing all of the muscles of the face. Once the body is in a more easeful state, connect to the feeling of your natural breath through the effortless movements of the belly, ribs, and chest and the feeling at the nose…lastly, finding your point of focus as you move into the next limb of practice.

Creating the Conditions for Pratyahara

Close your eyes and begin to allow your awareness that has been on outside world all day to slowly turn inward.

Begin to notice the current feeling of your physical body, just checking in with your current state. Then start to feel a softening of lower body...hips and legs completely releasing, sinking into the support beneath you.

*Continue to feel grounded and supported in lower body while, at the same time,
feeling the top of your head gradually reach up toward the sky, creating a feeling of length and openness in the spine.*

Allow the space of the shoulders to soften, feeling this softening flow down the length of the arms, pooling softness into the palms of the hands and fingers.

Begin to feel as if the collarbones start to widen horizontally to bring more expansion into the chest. Allow your lips to part, just a little bit, for a complete release of the jaw...even softening the lower row of teeth, relaxing the tongue, and feeling the whole mouth soften.

*Then notice the feeling of the roof of the mouth, the feeling of your soft palate...
allow the roof of your mouth to lift and widen, your soft palate to lift and expand as if you are in awe or witnessing something beautiful.
Feel this expansion move up through your sinuses, eyes, forehead, top of the head...*

Check with the space behind your eyes and forehead; observe the
current space of your mind. Then, just like in body, release any
unnecessary holding or tension in the space of your mind. Begin to
feel your space of mind gradually becoming
a little lighter, a little clearer, more open and spacious.
Continuing to allow your space of mind to stay in this opening,
clearing state, bring your mind's eye—your one-pointed focus—to
the feeling of your body naturally breathing.

Just notice the current rhythm of your belly,
the gentle expansion and release of the ribs,
the continuous rise and fall of chest,
the natural stream of breath entering and exiting the nose.

Dharana ~ Holding Focus

Once you are able to release the tug of the external world, the next
thing you will connect to is all of the dialogue and thoughts in your
mind. These are not arising because you are noticing them; they
are already there, clouding and getting in the way of everything
you experience and perceive in your life. This is the layer of your
wisdom, your intellect, the aspect of mind that judges, decides,
determines, and processes all of the information taken in through
the automatic mind of the senses. Just like all other aspects of this
inward journey, when you are able to bring your whole attention to
the space of your mind, it is like holding up a mirror to see your
current state and getting a front-row seat to your mental habits and
tendencies toward specific thoughts and stories. While this may
seem like a daunting task to so closely observe the state of your
mind, especially if it feels chaotic or full of clutter, by tuning in,
you become aware of all of the old thoughts that are unconsciously
taking up space and affecting how you experience life. The first
step to clearing the clutter and developing more clarity is *just
noticing it.*

Once you notice your mind full of thoughts, worries, and stories, it can feel very difficult to go any deeper into meditation. The next tool of practice and "rung of the ladder" helps you peel back the layer of distraction in your "thinking mind" so the dialogue in your mind space is no longer a disturbance to your focus. This is the yogic technique of *dharana,* holding concentration in one direction.[6] With this tool of practice, you are able to cultivate an effortless attention where your focus is not pushed or pulled by the thoughts in your mind. T.K.V. Desikachar describes this concept:

> Imagine a large reservoir of water used by farmers for watering their fields. There are channels leading away from the reservoir in different directions. If the farmer has dug all the channels to the same depth, the water runs equally in all directions. But if one channel is deeper than the others, more water flows through it. This is what happens in dharana: we create the conditions for the mind to focus its attention in one direction instead of dispersing in many different directions.[7]

This practice allows your single-processor mind to rest and gradually strengthens your ability to create this effortless attention with more ease. In the process of holding your focus, by releasing your grasp on the busy mind, your clutter of thoughts slowly starts to float farther away from your awareness, becoming less and less of a distraction until it no longer takes up space. This does not mean that you will completely forget memories that the thoughts are connected to, yet you gradually release the emotional coloring of the memories so that they no longer draw your awareness down the path of reliving the experiences these memories may have once created. Through the practice of *dharana,* you gradually clear up all of the unnecessary clutter clouding your perceptual view of experiencing life and gain a greater ability to be present in all moments. You have the ability to train your mind, like a muscle, to focus on one area and gain greater control over your thoughts so you are not unconsciously swept away with them. As you gain a stronger focus, your general concentration in all areas of life will become easier. You will be able to focus on what you are doing and be present in each current moment without busy thoughts of the mind being a distraction.

It is helpful to consider the scattered content of thoughts as "clutter" because when you notice old stories and dialogue in mind, it can feel very personal, real, and significant. Yet this is just an outdated collection of data mixed with whatever your perception and emotion was when you took in that information. It no longer needs to take up space or have any effect on your current perception of yourself, your life, or the world and people in it. Every moment, every breath, is a fresh beginning, an opportunity to grow by shedding anything you are grasping on to from the past that is not allowing you to experience this new present moment. The mind likes to associate, and you can develop a habit of comparing new information to what you already know or remember. Cleaning up your space of mind by loosening your unconscious grip on old mental perceptions and habits helps you avoid being distracted by previous thoughts, opinions, experiences, and emotions that cloud your experience. This enables you to perceive each thought in a new way, learn something from it, and then release it. This is not an analyzing process but a clearing process. In the clarity, you will be able to soften your mental grip, expand your view, and release all of the unnecessary clouding of your perception and understanding.

The practice of *dharana* is as simple as *bringing your focus to an object of attention,* noticing when your awareness has been drawn away by a thought stream, gently bringing it back to your point of focus, and continuing this process. This can feel difficult, so there are specific techniques you can utilize to help accomplish a single-pointed focus with more ease. One of the best objects of attention for your focus to rest upon is your breath...*the feeling of your natural, effortless breath.* It is portable, something that is always available to you at any moment. It is also the connection of your mind and body, the direct link the mind uses to connect to body and the body uses to respond back. It is the perfect tool at the start of your practice for drawing your awareness inward and is also the foundation of being able to deepen and expand on the practice. Tapping into the feeling of your body naturally breathing is a wonderful way to experience observing what is; without needing to do or try, your body effortlessly breathes. To connect to this, begin to notice the sensations of your body, check in with your physical state in stillness, and then start to observe the natural movement occurring in your body. As your lungs begin their inhale, your belly, ribs, and chest will gradually expand and, with your exhale, gradually deflate. You can also connect to the feeling and sensation of the breath at the nose.

Breath Awareness

Allow your body to soften, release, and become still. Then notice the gentle, effortless movement within that stillness, notice the feeling of your body naturally breathing...
the subtle movement of the belly, gentle expansion and release of the ribs, continuous rise and fall of the chest, even the feeling and sensation of your natural breath flowing in and out of the nose. Allow your awareness to just rest on this effortless, natural stream of breath at the nose. If a thought or outward distraction draws your mind away, as soon as you notice, gently bring it back to the stream of breath at the nose.

At times, the mind can find it difficult to just rest on the feeling of breathing, so you can add specific aids for focus to your breath awareness such as mantras, visualizations, and mudras. A *mantra* is a repetitive sound, word, or thought that can be used as our "object of focus".[8] Through this practice, you bring your focus to your natural breath and then add a simple word to this awareness, allowing the mind to rest on the flow of breath along with a subtle mantra. We will begin with a simple "reporting of the news," as Erich Schiffmann would say. Just reporting what you experience, with every inhale think *in* and with every exhale think *out*.

Mantra Meditation

Begin to observe the feeling of your body naturally breathing…
the current rhythm of the belly,
gentle movement in the front, back, and sides of the ribs,
subtle rise and fall of chest,
connecting into the feeling of natural breath, effortlessly flowing in and out of the nose.
Continuing to allow your awareness to just rest on the feeling of this stream of breath at the nose, add a silent mantra, a mental whisper…
with every natural inhale think "in," with every following natural exhale think "out."

If a tendril of thought or outward distraction draws the mind's eye away, as soon as you notice, gently bring it back to the feeling of breath at the nose…
in…out

Other simple mantras to utilize are:

I - Am
Throughout our lives, we *are* many things…we all wear many hats. This is a mantra to release all of those things and just sink, just ground into our being.

Sat - Nam

At times, a mantra with english words can create dialogue instead of helping us quiet it. In these cases, utilizing a Sanskrit mantra (which we do not have a dialogue connection to) can be helpful. This mantra translates to "I am," with nothing more afterward. This is simply another way to sink into your being.

So - Hum

This is another simple Sanskrit mantra that translates as "I am that," indicating you are one with all, forming a complete connection with no separation between yourself and all other living beings. It is also thought that if you could hear the subtle sound of your natural breath at the nose, it would make a soft *so* on the inhale and *hum* on the exhale, allowing you to connect deeply with the natural sound and rhythm of your breath.

Just like your mantra, you can also add a subtle visualization to your breath awareness. After resting your focus on the stream of breath, you can begin to envision this stream of breath navigating in a certain direction or serving specific needs in different areas of the body. These are all imagined through natural, effortless breathing.

White Light - Black Smoke

Allow your awareness to rest on the feeling of breath at the nose. Then visualize every natural inhale as a stream of white light, moving into the mind and clearing out space. With every following natural exhale, visualize a stream of black smoke ridding space of mind of what is no longer needed.

Area Behind the Navel

Allow your awareness to rest on the area behind the navel. Simply observe the natural rhythm of movement there.

Navel to Throat - Throat to Navel

Bring your awareness to the feeling of effortless breathing in the body. Then begin to imagine your natural inhale moving from the navel to the throat and your natural exhale moving from the throat to the navel. Continue to allow your awareness to rest on the natural movement of breath...navel to throat, throat to navel.

Alternate Nostril Visualization

Bring your awareness to the feeling of effortless breath at the nose. Then, on your next natural inhale, imagine the breath going into the right nostril, up to your third-eye point and then your natural exhale going from the third eye out through the left nostril. Observe the next natural inhale going into the left, up to third-eye point and your natural exhale going out through the right. Continue to visualize your effortless breath, alternating in and out of each nostril.
*You may also start on the left.

Another set of tools that can be utilized to enhance our focus are *mudras*. These are symbolic gestures often practiced with the hands and fingers that help facilitate the flow of energy within us as we are moving our focus inward.[9] Since our hands are a subtle reflection of the mind, if you notice grasping or disconnect in the mudra, it is a sign that the same thing is happening in the mind. In this way, the mudra is a tell of what is occurring in mind space as well as a gentle tool to help our focus stay soft and present.

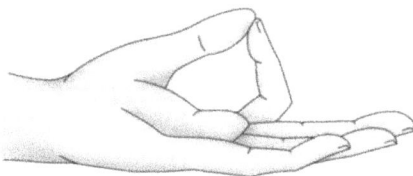

Gyan Mudra (Seal of Knowledge)
Touch the tip of the index (first) finger and the tip of thumb together, keeping your

44

other three fingers straight. This mudra stimulates knowledge, wisdom, receptivity, and calmness.

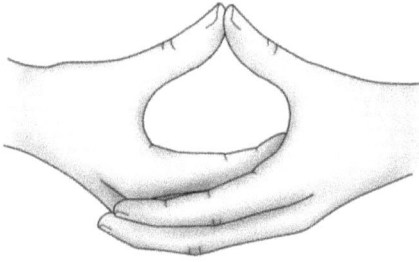

Dhyana Mudra

This is one of the most commonly known and widely practiced mudras, found across several religious and spiritual traditions. Rest your hands, palms facing up, on top of one another at the navel with your right hand on top, and place your thumb tips together to form a triangle.

In this mudra, the right hand, representing enlightenment and states of higher consciousness, rests over the left hand, representing illusion. This is believed to bring balance to the two sides of the body and brain as a means of quieting the mind. This technique improves your concentration, helping you progress from dharana toward deeper states of meditation, inner peace, and equanimity.

Dhyana ~ Meditative State

The next limb in our journey of practice is similar to *pratyahara* in the sense that it is not necessarily something we do but something that occurs when all of the conditions are right. When you are able to draw your awareness away from the distraction of your thoughts and senses by resting your one-pointed focus, this creates the conditions for the next rung of practice to occur. This limb is known as *dhyana* and is defined as "focus of attention in one direction, *binding consciousness to a single point.*"[10] This state of deep concentration creates the right conditions for you to shift into a meditative state.

It is when your focus is resting on one particular thing that all of the pulls and tugs of distraction cease so the movement of the mind can become less and stillness can rise. While all of the practices leading up to this help you glide into meditation with more ease, the previous limb of holding your focus (our dharana practice) is the most important step. Your focus must create an effortless connection to a particular object so that you can release activity of mind and just rest. It is this easeful connection that allows the mind to move into a state of meditation. Once this occurs, the practice of continuing to bring the mind back to your point of focus (dharana) is no longer needed; you can release your holding of focus and just sink into the stillness. If something does draw your focus away, utilize your object of attention to gently guide you back. Once the connection is made again, soften the hold of focus and sink back into the stillness. The practice of dharana helps you reach dhyana and is your path back if your awareness drifts in practice.

Once you reach the stillness, rest there and abide in this space…this *is* the practice of dhyana. This is accomplished through the release of all of the elements that brought you here; it is the destination and purpose of the practice to reach this level of stillness in the mind. Immerse yourself in this deep meditative state. Begin with five to ten minutes of silence, eventually allowing at least fifteen minutes or more for this portion of your practice.

Chapter 3

The Journey

Close your eyes and begin to allow your awareness,
that's been on outside world all day,
to slowly start to turn inward.

Observe the current feeling of your physical body...
notice the current feeling of your natural breath...
the current feeling of your space of mind...
the starting point of your practice.

Then allow your lower body to ground into the support beneath
you as the crown of your head extends to the sky.
Soften your shoulders, arms, palms of the hands,
then allowing for a subtle lift of the chest,
length in the neck and softening of the face.

Observe your awareness naturally tuning in to
the effortless rhythm of your body breath.
As you notice aspects of your environment tugging on your senses,
begin to draw your awareness inward to your point of focus.
Allow your awareness to rest there.
Continue to return there, sinking into a state of oneness with your
deepest self.

All of life is a journey as you continue to travel from moment to moment. In each of these moments, voyaging through the stages of your life, the scenery around you and the vehicle in which you are traveling shifts and changes. Maintaining a state of balance and health in all aspects transporting us through life makes us better equipped to experience the journey with clarity and ease. The limbs of yoga practice help us accomplish this, not only individually but also as a systematic process. When you use them in a specific sequence, they allow you to release the exact distractions you encounter on your journey. This is best explained through the understanding of the *koshas*—these are the five layers of your tangible and subtle body that cover the Self and make up the functioning system of your mind, body, and soul.[1] Collectively, they are the lens through which you view and experience your life.

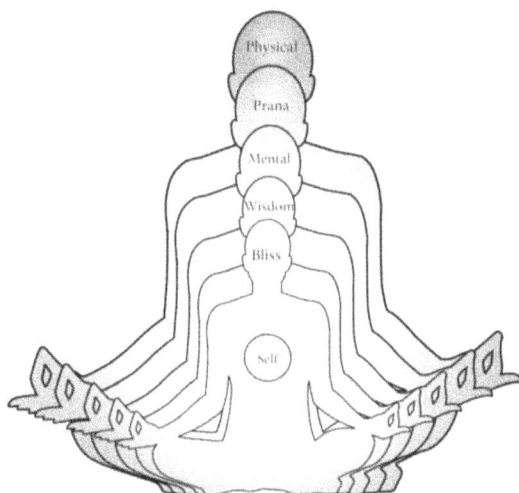

Figure 1. The Kosha Model

It is important to keep the koshas clear, open, balanced, and healthy since they interact with and affect one another, creating your experience of being alive. For instance, you could be in the most joyful, amazing moment, yet if you have pain in your body, feel energetically low, are distracted by your environment, or your mind is full of racing thoughts, you will not be able to experience the full delight of this moment. The obstacle of distraction within each of the layers of being can obstruct your perspective and ability to be present. Knowing how to access these individual layers of yourself is vital to caring for each aspect of your being as well as moving beneath the koshas to connect to your deepest self. Michael Stone eloquently describes this process:

> "The five kośas are a kind of magnifying glass or prism through which we can better understand the workings and interactions of perception, consciousness, feeling, breathing, and physiology. In addition, the kośas become a meditative tool through which we can undo the habits of the five kleshas… a set of strategies for how and where one should focus one's attention. This system offers a kind of sequential logic for meditative practice."[2]

These coverings are best imaged as layers of an onion in that you must peel back one to gain access to the next. We accomplish this by connecting to and releasing tension, holding, or blockages in each. The limbs of yoga practice help us to achieve this by offering tools that can be used in a specific order—like rungs of a ladder, each one helps us reach the next. The first layer of our being is the physical body, known as the *annamaya kosha*. Defined as a sheath that is nourished by food, it is our outermost layer, consisting of all physical form, and is also the layer that supports and sustains the others.[3] To help us keep it healthy and open so that it is not a distraction, we utilize the tool of asana, which allows us to nurture the body toward a state of comfort and stability so we can let go of it and our awareness can connect to the next kosha.

Next is the *pranamaya kosha*, layer consisting of prana, the energetic aspect that animates us and brings us to life.[4] It is the layer that connects the body and mind, as it is the life force that allows communication between the two. To move through this layer and keep it open and flowing, we can utilize pranayama techniques to help release any blocks or low-flowing prana that may be distracting us and impeding our ability to connect deeper. Once our prana is able to expand and flow more freely through us, we can connect to the third layer known as the *manomaya kosha*, the mind sheath.[5] This is the aspect of the automatic mind that includes the five senses. Whether we are intending to or not, we are constantly taking in information through the senses that the mind has to process. This is a lot of work, and it can be tiring for the mind to digest all that it is taking in. This outward distraction also makes it incredibly hard to connect any deeper in practice and in your life. Think of a time when you were looking for some relaxation or trying to meditate, yet the neighbor started mowing their grass or your dog began to bark, making it difficult to enter that relaxed state. Consider a time when you had a decision to make but were so busy in your daily life that you could not connect to how you truly felt. To move through this layer, we practice pratyahara, withdrawal of the senses. This technique keeps us from losing focus because of distractions in our environment.

When we are able to release the pull of the senses, we then connect to the next layer known as the *vijnanamaya kosha*, the wisdom sheath.[6] This is the aspect of the thinking mind, which decides, understands, and processes all of the data we are taking in from the outside world. It is important to be able to connect to this layer, as this is where we can access our deepest wisdom and insight. This is also where we find the unconscious tendencies and habits of the mind as well as old stories or internal dialogue (clutter) that we need to release. Yet this is not the final depth we can reach. Your true Self, the witness of life, is still beneath this layer of activity. While it is beneficial to be able to connect into this aspect of the mind, it is also a distraction for us to go any deeper, so we utilize the next limb of practice known as dharana. This technique of one-pointed focus (concentration in one direction) helps us peel back the layer of the wisdom sheath to enter the next kosha.

The fifth and final layer is the *anandamaya kosha*, the "bliss sheath." This is the innermost layer covering the Self, so it reflects its true nature. [7] Your deepest consciousness does not have any of the pain, emotions, or clutter that exist in the layers covering it. The true Self is pure; none of the suffering of human life exists within it, so once it is reached, the feeling of bliss can be experienced. This is the true feeling of *you*, the aspect of you that cannot be altered or changed, the aspect of you that is constant as opposed to the ever-changing physical body and mind. Once reached, you will be able to practice the next limb of yoga, which allows you to reside in this connection—the technique of dhyana (meditative state).

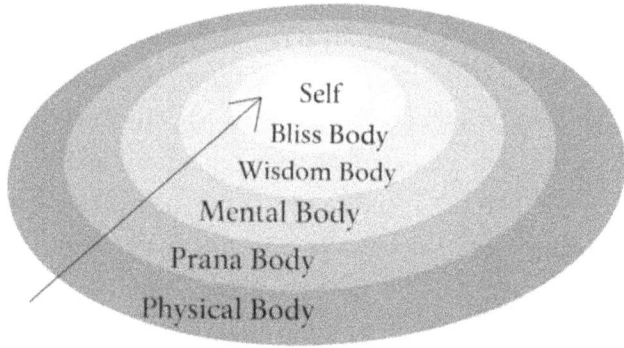

Self
Bliss Body
Wisdom Body
Mental Body
Prana Body
Physical Body

Figure 2. The Kosha Model

Map Inward

You can use your understanding of the koshas as a map for your journey inward, toward your peaceful center beneath distraction and thoughts, with the layers as your guide. The eight limbs of practice are your tools for the journey, specifically designed to help you each step of the way. With this knowledge, you not only have a more direct path to where you are going but also have an understanding of the way back through if something pulls you into a previous layer of awareness. For example, if you need to move or have an ache or itch that is distracting you, your awareness will come back to the body kosha. Similarly, you may notice a distraction in your pranic body if you take an active breath, if something occurs in your environment, or if a thought stream pulls you down a mental pathway. In each of these instances, your awareness will come back to that layer of distraction. Yet if it does, you know the way back. This does not mean you must use all of the techniques again; you just subtly go back the way you came—*consciously soften your body, observe natural breath, allow your senses to withdraw, and then return to your point of focus.*

Our Tools for the Journey

The limbs of yoga are amazing techniques that can be utilized individually and in a specific sequence, yet they are also practiced simultaneously. This is the origin of conceptualizing the yoga tools as limbs of a tree—each one grows as a result of supporting the growth of all of the others. While each step of the journey inward has a specific limb that is predominant, the limbs are also working in unison in the background in order for each technique to be performed. From the moment we close our eyes and start to tune in, we are beginning to cultivate the conditions for pratyahara. And then we continue this drawing inward, away from the pull of the senses, throughout our asana practice. While in asana practice, we are also utilizing pranayama, allowing our breath to be deep and full and our focus to unite with the feeling of breath and body. We guide our awareness inward as we find a comfortable posture and then move through a specific pranayama technique. While doing breathwork, there is a deep release of anything pulling the senses as our focus is immediately drawn toward the active breath. Then, as we release any doing and move toward simply observing a stable and easeful body, natural rhythm of breathing, and opening space of mind, we are allowing the other limbs to help us deeply cultivate the ability to turn the senses inward. This all serves the purpose of allowing our one-pointed awareness to rest on a specific point of focus. The individual limbs, each with their own importance, work incredibly well when implemented together as a step-by-step process to guide us toward an open, balanced system of being.

Clearing Process

With practice, we gain a greater ability to peel back and move beneath each layer. This process of connecting to and then softening our grasp to release the distraction is also a clearing process for each kosha. This is such an important process, as we perceive life from the depth we can access within. If you are not able to connect any deeper within yourself than your physical body, this is the view you experience life from. In this instance, you may feel as if your body is the totality of who you are, as if how you and others look is of the most importance, and your world may revolve around the physicality of all things. The process of peeling back that layer of awareness so that you can connect to deeper aspects of yourself is how you clear your perceptual view so you can experience life from a deeper state.

This process is the same for all layers of being. If you are not able to connect beyond your pranic layer, you experience life according to how it makes you feel, avoiding anything that has even a small possibility of being uncomfortable and utilizing— possibly to excess—things that make you feel good in the moment. Living in this state can create anxiety, loneliness, depression, and addictions. This also permeates the other layers of your being if you are not capable of releasing the distraction of the pull of your environment and going deeper than your automatic mind. Any outward distractions you are immersed in will encompass your perception of each moment of your life. Your interpretation of your life's events may then be overridden by whatever positive or negative elements you are exposed to. Lastly, if you are unable to go any deeper than your thinking mind, your entire experience of each moment will be determined by the opinions you form based solely on what you think you know. This mindset is a distraction from experiencing any new moments, feelings, and knowledge, which keeps you from growing, connecting, and truly seeing the beauty of your life and those in it.

Obstacles on the Journey

The tools we have reviewed help us move through the layers of the koshas with more ease as well as through greater obstacles we may encounter along the way. While these obstacles can vary, one of the biggest hurdles of practice is pain in the physical body. A much deeper and louder distraction than simple discomfort, pain can feel impossible to release, especially if it is intense or chronic. Meditating is an opportunity to reduce the intensity of our physical pain and find moments of relief as we begin to withdraw our awareness from body into deeper states of our being. Since the body is the first layer that we must release to gain access to our deeper states, the sensation of pain inhibits us from focusing on much else outwardly or inwardly. We will all endure pain at some point in our lives, so the ability to soften the hold it creates is greatly beneficial.

When practicing with physical pain, you approach each step in a softer way, meeting yourself where you are and gradually moving through the process from that point forward. Starting with your asana practice, the subtle postures and gentle movements allow you to release surface tensions and unconscious holding as well as the extra stress that naturally occurs when you hurt. Your breathing techniques allow you to bring your focus to something else—the feeling of breathing—and as you deepen and lengthen your breath, more prana will move into the spaces where tension is being released.

Next comes the most important aspect of practice for accomplishing physical release—pratyahara, where we create conditions to soften the pull of the senses. This is where we are able to disconnect from the distraction of pain that may be present in body by releasing the mind's connection to the sense of touch and feeling, withdrawing our focus from it. This is not a process of trying to suppress or stop the pain; it is a way of detaching your awareness from the pain. Just as if you hear the ticking of a clock when you start meditating only to realize at the end of your practice that you completely released your awareness of that sound, you can also release your awareness of physical pain and sensations. It is not that they go away (no one turned it off or removed the sound from the room) but that you are able to release your awareness and completely disconnect from it, or at least allow it to become softer and less distracting. As your senses gradually withdraw inward toward your point of focus, moving into a meditative state heightens your ability to maintain moments, or even extended periods, of disconnect and release.

The process of meditation practice helps us to experience this relief and also aids in reducing pain overall. Scientific studies on how the body and mind respond to pain have uncovered that, when there is pain in the body, there is an initial source followed by the body's and mind's reactions to it. These reactions can act as an intensity button for the suffering we endure. For instance, when there is pain in one area of the body, all muscles, tissues, and nerves are affected, which intensifies the pain throughout the entire body. With all of this, we start to hold our body and move a little differently, causing more misalignment and pain. The mind has a similar reaction to physical pain that heightens its intensity. As described by Danny Penman Ph.D. in *Psychology Today* online publication:

Pain comes in two forms: Primary and Secondary. Each of these has very different causes—and understanding this gives you far greater control over your suffering. Primary pain arises from illness, injury, or damage to the body or nervous system. You could see it as the raw information sent by the body to the brain. Secondary pain is the mind's reaction to Primary pain but is often far more intense and long-lasting. Crucially, it is controlled by an "amplifier" in the brain that governs the overall intensity of suffering.[8]

Secondary pain stems from the reactions that the body and mind have to the primary source, and it is through our practice that we are able to gradually soften the unnecessary holding and tension that arises in the body and the grasping of awareness in the mind to "turn off" this intensity button. As your body begins to release its grip, you will also start to notice misalignment occurring due to tension and gradually adjust. In this way, you are able to utilize your practice as an investigative tool for discovering a pain source and softening the physical effects it creates as well as eliminating the added reactions of your focus that magnify that pain.

There are many other obstacles we may encounter in our lives that seem to get in the way or distract us from practice, caring for ourselves, and staying balanced. We approach the practice and ourselves in the same way whether we feel energetically blocked or imbalanced, are carrying emotional pain, or feel mentally clouded or chaotic. In relation to our practice, these are all just obstacles or distractions in the path toward moving beneath them into stillness. Being able to release them, for even a moment, helps us to witness this more clearly. Another key component of our practice that allows us to release obstacles is one-pointed focus. Through the technique of dharana, your focus is able to connect to and rest on your object of attention without being distracted or pulled away from it. This is the aspect of practice that allows your senses to fully withdraw and release the connection. Swami J describes, "The senses are said to follow the mind in the same way the hive of bees follows the queen bee. Wherever she goes, they will follow. Similarly, if the mind truly goes inward, the senses will come racing behind."[9]

Reflecting on Your Life

When we strengthen the body through exercise, we start to feel stronger throughout the rest of the day. Similarly, when we are able to soften tension, release distractions, and focus during meditation, we become able to do this with more ease throughout our day. This ability does not start and end with practice; this is just where we learn to do it. What we experience in our practice we can also cultivate in our lives. Through practicing on the cushion, we also learn how to notice sources of imbalance and care for each aspect of ourselves in every moment of our everyday lives.

On a deeper level, once we are able to connect to and clear unnecessary tension and clutter from each kosha, we begin to see how much these layers interact. For example, if you are low in energy, your body will feel fatigued and your mind sluggish. If you hurt in your body, you can become energetically blocked, your mind only able to focus on the discomfort. What is occurring in one layer affects the whole. On the other hand, this is how you balance and clear each. Softening the body will allow prana to flow more freely, help your mind release tension, and so on. While the koshas include many individual components, the entire system determines *how you feel* and experience your life.

Another important aspect of this connection and clearing is that, once you experience the koshas as layers covering Self, this deters you from identifying with them or confusing them with who you truly are. You are not your physical body, as it will continue to shift and change. You are not how you feel at any given moment or even how you habitually feel about or respond to the world around you. You also are not your thoughts or the stories that you think you know about yourself. All of these aspects of your being do and will shift and change throughout your life. The aspect of your soul, the Self, the seer that can observe and witness all of this, never changes; that is you we are. The ability to see, connect, and observe your life from that perspective is key to experiencing yourself and the world around you with clarity and ease.

All of these benefits evolve gradually. Just as with anything else you are trying to cultivate in your life, it takes time and consistency. Consider a drinking glass that you use every day. If you never clean the glass, it will become very dirty. If you only clean it once in a while, it will be harder to clean and will be dirty most of the time. However, if you create a routine of cleaning the glass every day, it will remain clean and any dirt that collects will be noticeable. If you approach the care of your body and mind in this same way, you will achieve a similar outcome. There are no shortcuts, yet it is doable and attainable for every one of us to cultivate a clearer, more balanced state within by caring for ourselves and molding our being through new habits. Your body, energy, and mind are in a perpetual state of change, yet you have the ability to influence and guide the direction you are shifting toward and the quality of your state of being.

Chapter 4

Deepening the Connection

Connect into your environment, the space that surrounds you...
observe sounds in the distance,
sounds in this building,
sounds in this room...

Notice the feeling of the floor beneath you,
the sensation and temperature of the air against your skin.
Then allow your awareness to connect to
the current feeling of you...

Your physical body,
rhythm of your natural breath,
current state of your space of mind...
tapping into your inner environment,
then releasing any holding or tension in your whole being.

Allow your mind to expand by observing the feeling of
whole body breathing...
with each natural inhale, the whole body gently expands, becoming
a little lighter; with every following natural exhale, the whole body
deflates, grounding deeper into the support beneath you and
surrounding you.

As your view of meditation begins to expand, an understanding reveals itself that it is not just another thing you need to *do*, it is a means of cultivating a deeper relationship with yourself and an inward connection to how you think and interact with the world around you. It allows you to have a clearer understanding of who you are and how you are experiencing life. If, at times, you feel confused or disconnected, you can cultivate a clear path and view within. We all have the ability to do this—we just forget, are out of practice, or need to be reminded of the way. The path within gets cluttered as we live our lives and become easily distracted, yet our meditation practice helps us continue to clear the path and strengthen our focus. It is so important that you remember and develop this ability, as you are the only one who can understand and experience yourself in this way. You are the only one who will ever be able to get this close to your *Self*.

There is just one stipulation: you must *practice*. A weight will not strengthen a muscle if you just learn about how it will help or look at it from time to time; you must use it. If you use it in the right way, it will strengthen your muscles and you will be able to use them more efficiently. This same concept applies to your meditation practice. If you do it, you will cultivate the benefits. You can choose to only utilize these techniques every once in a while to relieve surface-level tension, but a shift will occur when you start to incorporate these practices into your daily habits and routines. This is when you begin to fine-tune and cultivate a *new norm* within yourself of balance and equanimity. Experiencing your life in this way, with this clearer perspective, allows you to see things how they truly are and know how you feel and think without the filter of old experiences, emotions, attachments, or irritability. This is extremely beneficial because stress, tension, mental clutter, and attachments to all of the distractions in life are patterns we start to fall into when we are always on the go, not aware or paying attention. The counterbalance to this mode of being is forming new habits that reverse this tendency.

In order to alter our habits to the extent that we are able to elevate our state of health and well-being, it is helpful to incorporate these practices every day. For example, if you wanted to improve your digestion and nutrition through your diet, eating a healthy meal once per week is not going to create much of a change. When you eat nourishing food, you take in the nutrients from them and feel the benefits; when you do not eat nourishing food, you do not receive the benefits. Your meditation practices nourish you in the same way. When you begin to incorporate them into your daily routine and cultivate new healthful habits is when you will truly experience the shift in quality of how you feel and operate in your life.

Broader Scope of Practice

From a strong foundation, you are able to grow and expand what you are cultivating in your practice into your life. Seated meditation has the deepest benefits, as it is the basis for connecting beneath all layers of distraction. It is where you will discover the ability to connect deeper, get better at it, and clean up space so you can continue living in that mode of clarity in all aspects of your life. Once you begin your practice, you will find there are more ways you can subtly connect to this softening and opening experience of life when off the cushion. Erich Schiffmann describes, "There are three ways to meditate…in seated posture, in asana (which includes walking, laying down, all postures of body), and then all the rest of the time."[1] For example, there are many different fruits and each one has different benefits. Bananas, apples, and oranges, while all fruit, each offer different nutrients and nourishment. This also applies to our practices, which are all wonderful and beneficial, yet in different ways.

Seated meditation, in silence and stillness with eyes closed, is a vital way to practice, as it removes the many distractions of movement, sight, and other sensory input, creating an opportunity to experience a deeper release of tension and connection inward. Yet we can also find this connection and be fully present when moving the body through asana or on a mindful walk outdoors. We do this by uniting our awareness with the movements of body, finding stability and ease within, and drawing our focus to the feeling of breath so as not to be distracted by thought. We can also bring this mindfulness into whatever we are doing, such as being completely present while washing dishes, creating art, having a conversation, or in a simple everyday moment.

What you discover in your practice is reflected in your life, and what you learn in your life shows up in your practice. Both intermingle to represent the totality of practice; there is no separation. The remaining limbs of yoga help us expand into the broader scope of practice as we begin to utilize the eight aspects of practice beyond seated meditation. It is helpful to introduce the practices of yoga with the limb of asana since the body is the first layer of being that we experience life through and the first thing we connect to when we close our eyes and draw our awareness inward. Yet once we start to practice asana and the following limbs of yoga, it is also essential to learn and practice the first two limbs of the *yamas* and the *niyamas*. They naturally begin to develop alongside the other techniques, yet consciously practicing them is the fundamental foundation for growth and experiencing the full benefits of practice. To be able to turn inward and experience a peace and calm within, it is important to have an easeful connection with your environment and those in it as well as with yourself. These first two yogic practices help to strengthen your relationship with the world and with yourself, creating a stable foundation for thriving in your practice and in your life.

Yamas ~ *how we connect with the world around us*

The first limb of yoga helps you unite your awareness with your relationship with the world around you,[2] offering tools that bring clarity and balance and prevent any disconnect or unrest from being an obstacle to the mind in practice and living. Your connection to your environment is of the utmost importance, as it is the space you reside in, the energy you are immersed in every day. Without feeling a sense of ease in your relationship with the outer world, you will not have the stable foundation needed to truly flourish and grow in your practice and your life. Practice of the *yamas* is the first step to cultivating a greater connection to your environment. This limb consists of five behaviors and interactions with all other living beings.

Like the other limbs, it is a practice. The yamas are not about how we currently feel about the world and people around us. They help us connect, especially when we may not feel like it. For example, asana is not only good for you when you already feel stable and easeful; it is a technique to meet your body where it is and guide it to that state. The yamas are helpful in that same capacity. We do not practice because we already feel united; we practice so that we can create this state. Through a deeper understanding and clarity of your personal connection to the world as a whole, you can positively fine-tune your interactions and behaviors with your environment and those in it. Similar to when you may feel tension in the body and the postures help you connect to its source and release it, the yamas can help you alleviate feeling completely disconnected due to the pain, suffering, and distress in the world. You may also feel, at times, as if it is impossible or undesirable to connect with those in your immediate workplace, family, or community and beyond. This is when these practices come into play. They help to unite your awareness of your own actions, behaviors, and responses to your environment with practices that lead you toward a more balanced understanding. It does not necessarily mean you will begin to feel a positive connection, accept negative actions, or change others' behaviors. These practices simply allow you to become aware of the disconnect and refine your behaviors toward others in order to shift your perception and establish an undistracted environment in which you can reside.

The limb of the yamas consists of five aspects of practice. The first of these is non-violence, or *ahimsa*.[3] This practice encompasses all actions—physical, mental, and emotional—

toward all living creatures. We can implement this practice by consciously acting with kindness and thoughtfulness toward all we encounter. We begin by allowing our actions throughout the day to be mindful and considerate to others. Eventually, this will become more effortless and how we naturally interact with the world. When we start to feel balanced and find more clarity of mind, the separation between us and all other living things seems to dissipate. Through this, we start to feel in harmony with others and recognize our connection with the living world around us.

The second aspect connects us to truthfulness, or *satya*,[4] with our words and actions. This practice encompasses our behaviors, speech, and intentions. While we should refrain from speaking the truth if it would cause negative consequences, create conflict, or be harmful to another, when we are able to live in a personal environment of truth and authenticity, it helps us see others for "the light they truly are" and allows them to see the same in us. This concept is similar to the intention behind the gesture and phrase "*namaste,*" translated as "the light in me honors the light in you."[5] This salutation is typically used at the end of class for those who have practiced alongside us, paired with a slight bow and hands together at heart center. To develop this tool of the yamas, you observe our own thoughts and actions that may not be aligned with your truth or the reality of a situation. Notice if there are deeper emotional attachments that may be creating delusions surrounding what is true for you. Most aspects of false perceptions arise from unprocessed fears or negative emotions from previous experiences that cause us to avoid seeing the truth. There are also instances when we are aware of what is true yet hold back or speak untruths due to the same source of fear. In both instances, the key is to bring clarity to your mind and trust yourself to experience the reality of the moment without allowing your fear to diminish your connection with the world around you. We are all connected.

The next practice of the yamas is through non-stealing, or

asteya.[6] While this does refer to the taking of actual objects that do not belong to us, this practice also includes theft of others' time, energy, information, work, ideas, and so on. The urge to take from others typically arises from feelings of inadequacy, unhappiness, or lacking. The first step in asteya is to bring our awareness to any unconscious stealing in our lives and not only cease these habits but also implement a routine of giving. Cultivating a state of being that is abundant by selflessly contributing to the needs of others will create a state of balance and inner fullness with no need to take from anything outside of ourselves—we are complete.

In addition, there is the practice of non-excess, or *brahmacharya*,[7] which helps us conserve our energy so we do not feel depleted from our interactions with the world around us. In this context, excess refers to not only tangible items but also the activities we do, thoughts we have, stimulation or avoidances we seek…any and all things in our lives that utilize our time, senses, and energy. We can develop a pattern of swinging between states of intensity and fatigue when we are working hard, overstimulated, or running on overdrive and then crash. With this aspect of practice, we learn to utilize our energy in a balanced manner so as to avoid depletion. If your interaction with your environment and the people in it drains your energy to the point of hindering how you operate in this world, you will not have the energy you need to be present and connected to those in your life.

This practice also allows us to avoid unnecessary dependence on things that feed our senses but do not nourish us on a deeper level or cultivate lasting joy. These teachings describe how taking a balanced approach of moderation, between excess and elimination, helps us create fulfillment and find peace. We begin this practice by observing our current habits and routines. Most of the time, it is fairly easy to identify areas of your life where more balance is needed. It is the next step that is key: gradually reducing the habitual actions and thoughts you utilize too frequently in your daily routines while gradually incorporating elements that are lacking yet would nurture your being and propel you toward a more balanced state. The practice is to notice these patterns and then gradually adjust them in the direction of balance.

Lastly, the yamas include the practice of non-possessiveness, or *aparigraha*.[8] This brings us back to the concept of non-attachment as we begin to notice our grasping of the world around us. The practice begins with noticing our attachments to expectations and the actions of others. Grasping on to these ideals creates disappointment and disconnect with those around us. This also refers to our thoughts, stories, ideas, and emotions that affect how we perceive our environment. If we have a strong grip on these, any shift or change will create a sense of unease and prevent us from living harmoniously with the flow of life.

The yamas can be practiced on a small or large scale. The first step is to become aware of any actions, words, or even thoughts that are not in line with these practices; the next step is to gradually begin implementing them in your life. T.K.V. Desikachar describes what happens when the yamas become part of a person's daily life. He states, "For example, the more ahimsa—kindness and consideration—we develop, the more pleasant and friendly feelings our very presence engenders in others. And if we remain true to the idea of satya, everything we say will be truthful…For those who are always truthful, there is no difference between speech and actions—what they say is true. The *Yoga Sutras* also states that a person who is firmly anchored in asteya will receive all the jewels of this world. Such a person may not be interested in material wealth, but they will have access to the most valuable things in life." He continues to describe how if we have deep trust, we will have more energy and vitality, releasing our want of material possessions, and have more time to spend on living a balanced life.[9]

Niyamas ~ *how we connect with ourselves*

The second limb is known as the *niyamas* and consists of practices to help unite you with yourself and your inner world.[10] It includes five personal techniques to help you nurture self-awareness by eliminating obstacles to a deeper connection with yourself. Timothy Burgin of Yoga Basics describes, "The practice of niyamas helps us maintain a positive environment in which to thrive and gives us the self-discipline, humility, and inner-strength necessary to progress along the path of yoga."[11] While the first limb aims to bring you a balanced connection with your outer world, the term *yamas* is defined as "restraints;" therefore, to allow a boundless ease of being in your environment, you practice *not doing* behaviors that may hinder this connection. On the other hand, *niyama* is defined as "observances or behaviors," so these are the activities or habits that you must *do* to cultivate a deeper connection with your inner environment that influence how you see and experience life.[12] The practice of the niyamas brings your awareness to that which you must *do* to cultivate this clear connection. Then the other limbs give you tools to implement them.

This practice begins with the concept of cleanliness, or *saucha*.[13] This encompasses the cleanliness of the physical and energetic body as well as of the mind and thoughts. When your body and mind are free of toxic elements, you naturally function with ease, your energy moves freely, and your mind is able to connect inward. You can achieve this by making a conscious effort to make everything that you take in and digest from your environment be in its purest, cleanest form—food through your digestive tract, air through your lungs, products through your skin, and all of the information your mind takes in through the senses. By doing this, you can reduce the harmful side effects of non-nourishing food and unhealthy environments or thoughts. As you gradually lessen the unhealthy clutter you take in, it is also important to include cleansing practices to rid the body and mind of impurities currently present that you have unconsciously absorbed. The other limbs of practice will help you continue to cleanse and purify your being and develop a state of clarity in body and mind.

The next aspect is the practice of contentment, or *santosha*,[14] which helps you create an inner state of deep peace by releasing your attachments to "desires" that do not allow you, as Erich Schiffman would say, to be truly present in your "now moment." In this release, you can immerse yourself in gratitude for all that you have, allowing happiness and joy to live in the present rather than viewing it in light of the past and what was or the future and what could be. In this state, you still move forward toward goals, learn from experiences, and grow your understanding of life while preserving your sense of fulfillment from all you already have in the present moment. You begin to learn and experience this through your asana and pranayama practices as they help you to start the release of physical and energetic holds, enabling you to tap into your grasping of attachments. Then the practices of withdrawing the senses allow the mind's eye to rest and glide into a meditative state. It is here that you can continue to discover unconscious holding in mind space and gradually release your grip. Through your practice of the eight limbs, you are learning to sink into present moment and ungrasp all things distracting you from it. A sense of peace that arises as this occurs in practice helps you continue to cultivate this experience throughout the rest of your life. You can also cultivate a practice of gratitude for all that you have, look for the joy in every "now moment," and see opportunities for growth in any obstacles you may encounter.

The niyamas also include the practice of self-discipline, or *tapas*, meaning commitment to a practice.[15] This aspect represents the backbone of the practice and your ability to cultivate any of its benefits in your life. Simply learning about them does not have much effect on you. It is the doing, putting them into practice, that gradually allows you to shift into a more balanced and easeful state of being. This is not a discipline of struggle, an unenthusiastic effort, or a forceful endeavor. Through the practice of tapas, you are allowing your passion for your personal growth and development to be the driving force of your commitment to practice and releasing the suffering that can occur through living. This does not necessarily mean there will not be difficult moments or feelings of unease as you move through the journey, yet even when obstacles occur along the path, your dedication to yourself and the practice will allow you to overcome and persevere. The word *tapas* is also defined as "fire,"[16] indicating it is through our practice of self-discipline that the techniques illuminate the impurities in mind and body and help us burn them away. Tapas are the activities you can do to transform and purify your mind and body by keeping them healthy and clean, releasing the old and making room for the new, to create and strengthen positive habits and state of being. Your practice of tapas is how you grow in your practice and in your life.

The next aspect of the niyamas is self-study, or *svadhyaya*. This is the practice of inquiry and self-examination toward understanding the true nature of Self. *Sva* is defined as "self; the human soul" and *dhyaya* as "concentration or contemplation."[17] This practice helps you connect to and understand yourself through the process of self-discovery. It is a practice of taking a closer look inward at what you are and what you are not as well as how you hold tension, clutter, impurities, old cycles, and habits. It is not an analysis of the self but rather a practice of observing and discovering the deepest, oftentimes hidden, aspects of yourself. This is accomplished through the study of concepts in sacred yoga texts and then applying this knowledge of the whole of consciousness toward understanding your own individual consciousness.

The last aspect of this limb is the practice of surrender, or *ishvara pranidhana*, the practice of releasing your grip on needing to control, accomplish, or act in order for things to occur. *Ishvara* translates as "all-pervading consciousness" and *pranidhana* as "to surrender."[18] This is the practice of softening and releasing into the divine energy of all life and all that is beyond us and trusting the connection between the deepest aspect of yourself and this universal energy. It is a release of even the most ingrained tendencies to want to control outcomes, situations and others. It is surrendering to something bigger than ourselves, expanding our understanding of life beyond our immediate experiences and control. Immersing ourselves in the ultimate reality of life teaches us a deep sense of trust in self and the universe. It is a feeling of casting aside your burdens or the weight you are carrying around, a feeling of relief and freedom.

This practice can be considered the easiest one to implement, as the only effort required is to simply release and let go. While this seems like a simple task, our grasping can be intense and multilayered, having taken much time to cultivate; therefore, some find it to be the most difficult practice to accomplish. However challenging it may be, cultivating a clear path within and connecting to your deepest Self is one of the most important practices you can master. It begins with the awareness of your current grasping to control outcomes, then moving toward gaining a deeper trust in yourself, in divine energy, and in the process of life that naturally unfolds through simply moving in the direction of your goals. You can bring this into your days by finding gratitude for each moment and gradually releasing any fear that arises as you are learning to let go. Your asana and pranayama techniques will also help in this process; when you are able to release tension in body and energy, your mind follows suit and lets go as well.

Just as each limb of practice gives us the tools to put the niyamas into action and effect change, they also help our *layers of being* not be a distraction or obstacle to living life with clarity and ease. For example, asana practice allows you to check in with the current state of your body and soften unconscious tension that may be present. We are often unaware of how we naturally hold our bodies throughout the day, though unconscious habits of misalignment and tension can create unnecessary pain and discomfort. Your asana practice expands beyond just your movements on the mat to finding a stable and easeful seat on the cushion. While these are the core elements of the practice where you learn to connect inward and adjust, the word *asana* is simply defined as "posture, or to be established in a position."[19] Therefore, once you experience and understand how to find stability and ease in the position in which you hold your body in practice, you can bring these elements into your posture at any time. Your practice is where you learn and experience, and each practice helps to develop a more balanced way of living.

This also applies to our pranayama practice. These techniques help us learn how to connect into the current state of our prana within and then release unnecessary holding and restricted flow that lead to unease. You learn and develop these techniques on your cushion in the sequence of practice, yet once you know how to do this, it is a skill that is available to you at any time. At any given moment, you can tap into your current state and utilize a simple, deep, full breath (or more specific technique) to alleviate energetic holding or blockages and allow prana to flow more freely through your body. The benefits of our yoga practice continue to become integrated with our daily lives. Once we learn how to gradually withdraw our senses in our pratyahara practice, we get better at not allowing the distractions of the senses to draw us away from being present and mindful in our everyday moments.

Our dharana practice may be the one that has the largest impact on the positive shifts we start to experience in ourselves. This practice of strengthening our ability to focus on one object allows us to access this ability all of the time. It is the ultimate tool for developing the skill of naturally settling the mind and being truly present in all moments of life. This allows us to gradually cultivate a new baseline for how we perceive and experience life. As you learn how to do this on the cushion, you can also implement this technique in other aspects of your life—for instance, consciously trying to be more mindful throughout your day by simply concentrating on one thing at a time. When you eat, *just* eat; when you walk, *just* walk. Focus purely on what you are doing at any given moment. Just as in your sequence of practice, utilizing this technique will help you feel at ease in all of the quiet moments of life, enjoy the pauses in between all of the doing and being, and create a calm, peaceful mind space to clearly witness your true Self and your connection with the world around you.

Samadhi ~ *ultimate union*

There is one final tool of the eight limbs of yoga we have yet to discuss. This is the technique of *samadhi,* translated as "to bring together, to merge."[20] Just like our pratyahara and dhyana practices, this is not something we necessarily do; it is something that occurs when all of the conditions are right. Through your asana and pranayama practices, you are able to create conditions for the mind to release the pull of the senses and allow your focus to find an object of attention. Through the practice of returning your focus to the object, you are able to release the pull of thoughts, allowing your mind to move in a continuous flow with the object. Once you are able to merge into this meditative state and abide there with ease, your focus and the object begin to absorb into one another, allowing you to enter a state of samadhi. This is not a permanent state but a view that shifts your perspective and changes how you witness yourself and your environment.

Imagine you are living in a tiny town, not aware of anything or anyone further than what is in your community. Then, one day, you climb a mountain and are able to see that all around you are other small towns with streets, people, and animals just like yours. You also see how water flows through one town to get to yours and then from yours to another. You notice how the green landscape flows throughout all the land, almost making it seem like one large community. Once your view of life expands to an understanding of others moving through their lives in the same way, even when you return to your small street, you will still see the interconnectedness of the world. If you continue climbing the mountain and taking in the view, you will begin to experience this connection more and will continue to expand your view. This is how the practice of samadhi cultivates subtle clarity in how you experience your life. Through your practice of the eight limbs, in the sequence to release the obstacles of the koshas and reach your deepest layer, you are able to arrive in a state of samadhi and experience the connection and union of all. Similar to the other limbs of practice, samadhi is not a singular technique; it is an expansive state of being that, when achieved, allows you to practice within it. When you first begin to experience samadhi in your practice, it is a heightened state of clarity, just a subtle presence of thought, and a deep sense of connection. As you continue to practice, it begins to expand beyond this into a state where the concept of form or appearance of thought is released. This is when the point of connection between you and the object of meditation shifts to an experience of deep union and oneness with all. Michael Stone describes this experience as "the embodied vividness of nonseparation."[21] Just as when climbing the mountain, once experienced, your view of all life around you expands and you are able to vividly witness the connection of the whole living world and you in it. You are a part of the whole; the whole is a part of you. The invisible walls that once seemed to separate the two are gone, and what is left is *one*ness along with compassion that extends beyond yourself and your immediate environment to all living beings.

Chapter 5

Intertwining of Our Being

Body ~ Prana ~ Mind

Allow your body to settle and relax.
Begin to feel your whole body soften and release.

Observe the feeling of your body naturally breathing.
Then gradually begin to deepen each inhale and lengthen each
following exhale,
eventually allowing each inhale to completely fill the lungs with air
and each exhale to completely release every last drop.

Then begin to release all doing of the breathing.
Allow the breath to return to its natural, effortless pace.

Once again, tapping into the feeling of your body naturally
breathing, rest your awareness on this natural rhythm.

Every moment of each day, your body, mind, and the energy moving through them are always communicating with and affecting one another. They are separate yet can only function as a united system. Often, you are most aware of this connection through its negative effects. For example, if you are feeling mentally imbalanced, your body and energy will reflect this, and if your body is unwell or your energy is not flowing freely, it will influence the mind. Yet you can positively affect this connection as well by bringing balance to the body, energy, and mind in your practice. All of your yoga practices help to unite these three aspects of being to create a stronger union between them. As you find more steadiness and ease in the body, the mind begins to release and become more stable as well. Any tension in body and mind will gradually loosen, allowing your energy to flow more freely as you start to expand the prana within you through deepening and lengthening your breath. With this heightened prana, clarity will arise in the mind and your body will operate in a more balanced flow. As your mind begins to focus and become less distracted, your physical and energetic body will begin to release unconscious holding and tension, allowing the system as a whole to operate with more balance and ease. This is a continued lesson on the power you actually have to affect how you feel at any given moment. The practice of yoga is a science on how to balance these three aspects of our being. By practicing, we are able to gain deeper insight into where and what may need extra attention and learn specific tools of asana, pranayama, and meditation to help nourish and balance each. This balancing of the three also comes simply as the byproduct of practice—what occurs, what starts to cultivate within, and the outcome of daily practice incorporating the teachings, tools, and techniques of yoga into your daily life, cultivating new positive habits of living and being.

House for Our Soul

No matter how amazing your surroundings are in life, it is how your body feels (in health, balance, ease, and wellness) that is the place from which you experience all of life. Your physical body is the literal home for your soul during your time on Earth, so keeping it clean, uncluttered, and working well allows you to experience all of life in a clear, balanced way. Just as you clean and tidy your house, tending to things that need to be adjusted or mended to keep the heat working, the lights on, the structure stable enough for you to be protected from the elements, and so on, these same aspects apply to how your body provides you with a peaceful, clean inner environment and sustains your daily functioning in life. In the teachings of the koshas, this outermost layer of our being, annamaya, consists of all aspects of the physical form. This layer brings the others to life, as it is the tool we use to *do, connect, express, and interact* with anything in the physical world. The main aspects of the physical body that affect how we feel and function are our bones for structural support, muscles that move the bones, fascia that holds it all together, and the organs. These combined are the core physical components that influence how everything else works and feels. Due to this, it is imperative that you care for and nurture your physical self through practices that cultivate alignment, strength, and release, consciously avoiding toxic elements in your diet and environment as well as including more of those that nourish your physical self.

Life Force

Prana is that which creates movement in all living things, as it is the vital force that animates all of the living world.[1] Prana is the energy moving through the growing trees, the flying birds, your pumping heart, your expanding lungs, the reach of the senses, and all of the workings of the mind—thoughts, emotions, and so on. It is the force behind our ability to move, connect, and communicate with one another. In the map of the koshas, prana within us lies in the layer of being between the physical body and layers of mind, or pranamaya. This layer holds together the layers of body and mind and allows them to move and work together.

Within the human body, there are five main aspects to how this life force moves within us, each with a specific direction of flow. These forms of prana are known as *vayus,* or "winds,"[2] that work in different areas of the physical body and are the forces behind the vital functions located there. While each of these play a specific role, they must also work well as a system, in harmony with one another, for health and wellness in all areas of our being. When considering how you *feel* at any given moment, you are at your best and most balanced when all of your systems are flowing

76

freely and working well. If any are out of balance, whether sluggish, overactive, or blocked, it will begin to affect all of the others and how you operate. One of the specific aspects of prana, known as *udana-vayu,* dwells in the area of the throat and regulates the function of speech. Translated as "that which carries upward," this force manages our capacity for expression, growth, and confidence. If not flowing well, speaking, breathing, or throat difficulties may arise as well as an inability to express yourself. *Vyana-vayu* is the aspect that disperses energy throughout the body. It is defined as "outward moving air" and is the force that moves from our center out to all other parts of the body and is the force behind all of the circulation processes. The next is *samana-vayu,* which is located at the navel and translates as "balancing air." It is the force behind all digestion of food, experiences, thoughts, and everything else we take in from our environment.[3]

While the word *prana* represents the life force that is moving through the whole living world, another one of the specific expressions of that energy is known as *prana-vayu.* Defined as "forward moving air," this force resides in the chest area and is associated with inhalation as well as all inward and upward energy movement within the body. This aspect of prana within us also helps to direct and nourish the other four vayus. Lastly, there is the aspect known as *apana-vayu,* defined as "the air that moves away." It resides in the lower abdomen, extending into the pelvic floor,[4] and is associated with exhalation as well as regulating digestion and elimination of all things. It is the downward and outward movement of energy that, when out of balance, can create feelings of anxiety and desire for attachments in addition to weakness in the lower body or issues with the organs of elimination. These final two aspects are the main vayus (as they regulate all that enters and leaves the body) and can be tapped into directly through our breath. To allow the system as a whole—as well as each individual flow—to function in an open and balanced way, it is important to have an abundance of prana flowing throughout.

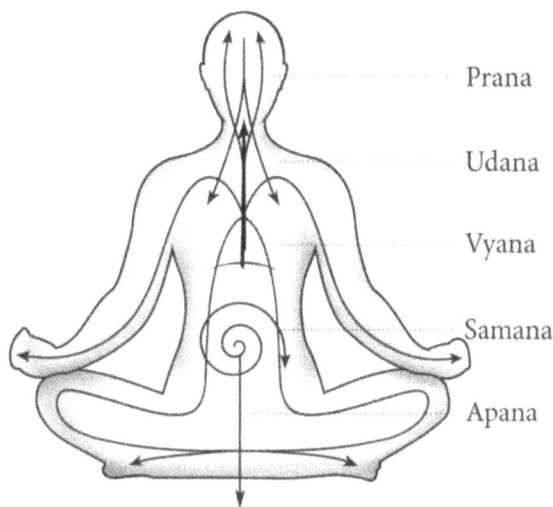

The Vayus

Labels on figure: Prana, Udana, Vyana, Samana, Apana

Consciousness

The aspects of mind, body, and energy are all things that are in our ever-changing environment and can be witnessed. While, at first, we may connect soul and consciousness as one, we can also witness the conscious mind. That which is witnessing, your innermost Self, your soul, the seer and observer of the mind and body, is known as *atman*.[5] The five layers of the koshas cover the soul, and your conscious mind functions through them, creating mind-body awareness and connection. This moving consciousness is known as *chitta*.[6] It is your ability to perceive and take in information as well as to process the thoughts of your inner world. It is the "totality of mind space" yet also the force behind all of its functioning. This is where and how we store past memories, emotions, thoughts, images, and impressions that we accumulate throughout our lives. It is the consciousness that allows us to be aware of it all, and—within this—arise the aspects of the sensory mind of *manas*, the intellect known as *buddhi*,[7] and the sense of a unique self called *ahamkara*.[8] These four components of the conscious mind, the senses, intellect, and identity are always working together. Imagine you are outside on a beautiful spring day. It is through chitta that you are able to be aware of this experience. Within that consciousness, through manas, you hear the birds, smell the blooming flowers, see the clear blue sky, and feel the warm breeze against your skin. Once this occurs, buddhi determines what this sensory information is and then, through ahamkara, connects to memories, past experiences, and how you feel and think about it. This process of the senses, intellect, and identity collaborating within awareness is continuously happening in each moment of your conscious day.

While your conscious mind is able to connect and work through all of the koshas, it is specifically through the manomaya kosha (layer composed of mana/mind) that you take in information from the outside world through the senses and specifically through the vijnanamaya kosha (layer composed of intellect) that you are able to understand, decide, and differentiate what is taken in. Your sense of identity can function through either of these two koshas, with each having a more positive or more negative effect on your self-worth and perspective of yourself. When your perception of identity is working through the manomaya kosha, it is filtered through memories, habits, and mental impressions of what you have previously experienced or been told. Yet when you are able to witness yourself through the vijianama kosha, your sense of identity is derived from observing and understanding yourself through intellect. In this way, you are able to learn and experience new possibilities about yourself as you release old dialogue surrounding what you previously believed to be true. Just as we want the body's systems to work well and all aspects of the pranic body to flow freely, it is important that all components of the conscious mind are operating in harmony.

Creating Balance

Your body, mind, and quality of prana within are always shifting, yet through your yoga practices, you have the ability to move these changes in a positive direction toward balance. You are able to cultivate stability and ease in your physical body through all of the various types of yoga asana. In each posture, you bring your body toward a greater state of alignment. While all of our bodies are built differently, the baseline structure is the same. The purpose of asana is to bring your current state toward this structural foundation of alignment so that you create a physical state of ease and stability. The key elements that distinguish an asana from just moving or being in your body are the same elements that allow this shift toward structural stability and ease to occur. As you allow your awareness to tune inward to how the body currently feels and then move through postures that specifically bring you toward balance, you learn how to detect misalignment and use postural tools to shift back toward center.

There are different ways to approach the practice of asana. Our active postures help us to stretch and strengthen the muscles while we move the bones toward alignment. We can also utilize seated, supine, and prone postures by releasing long holds to target the fascia surrounding muscles and bones. This connective tissue is thought to be where the meridians, or energy lines, of the body are, so keeping it soft and supple is helpful to how we feel physically and energetically. We can also approach posture in a supported way to deeply relax the body to the extent of allowing the nervous system to move into rest-and-restore mode by activating the parasympathetic nervous system. When we feel aligned and balanced in physical body, prana can flow more freely through us.

For a detailed description of these styles of asana practice, see Chapter 7.

Through our pranayama techniques, we increase the amount of prana within us. When the body, especially the fascia, is open and subtle, this higher quality of prana flows freely through us and helps the process of releasing unconscious holding or tension. This understanding reveals that, while at times we may think we have no control over how we feel, we actually have the ability to change and positively shift our current state of being by creating an unobstructed flow of high-quality prana within the body through our asana and pranayama practices. By doing this, we not only have the ability to feel better and improve the functioning of the body but can also elevate state of mind, as it is directly linked to the quality of prana within us. Through this, we have the ability to feel and function better not only in body but also in state of mind, as it is also closely linked to the quality of prana within us. When our prana is low, we feel restless, confused, cloudy, or stuck in mind. When our prana is high, we feel peaceful, balanced, light, and vibrant in mind. Since we can influence the flow of prana through the flow of breath, we have the ability to shift the way we feel energetically, physically, and mentally at any moment as well as on a daily basis to cultivate a new baseline of living.

When it comes to prana and chitta, they are both streams of energy and are oftentimes described as two aspects of the same stream.[9] This is why they have such a strong effect on each other and why you tend to bring your point of focus to natural breath in your asana and meditation practices. When you bring your consciousness to the prana moving through you, it allows them to unite and reconnect. Michael Stone describes, "We are trying to bring these two streams closer and closer together. The paradox is that the two streams are always fundamentally intertwined but our distracted mind keeps pulling them apart."[10] The combination of the two allows you to be a living conscious being; in this way, they are one. They also have many distinct functions and responsibilities that draw them away from each other. If you are predominantly operating in the mode of continual distraction of the environmental pull of senses and the thinking mind, you are not allowing for moments when these two streams of energy can unite, and then a disconnect can occur.

Your meditation practice allows you to reunite your conscious mind with the flow of breath; due to this reunion, a positive ripple starts to emerge. When the flows of energy are not being separated, they work in unison toward a common goal. Imagine having an hour for lunch in between meetings to eat, digest, and rest. It has been a busy morning, and you need to nourish yourself and pause in order to move through your afternoon with clarity and ease. Yet, instead, you eat quickly while walking around, talking, or dabbling on your computer. Due to the rush, your food did not digest well and no time was allowed to release all of the doing of mind. The goals of nourishment of body, rest of mind, and energetically resetting were not achieved because of not allowing the three to reset and reconnect. This is a tangible example of how peace of mind and ease of being are difficult to achieve without the redirection of the unified stream of conscious mind and prana within. When all forces are moving toward a desired goal of balance within a stable and easeful body, harmony and well-being can be achieved.

These positive ripples not only affect the current moment but also help the forces of mind, body, and prana work together consistently, in every moment. Through this, we are able to release the habitual grooves of imbalanced functioning. When energy can flow through the body without being obstructed by habits of distraction, the mind can settle and the trio of our being can find balance. We then begin to experience how the body, mind, and flow of prana can be positively transformed through practice, releasing that which cultivates imbalance while gradually molding a new way of being. Just as when you strengthen your physical body you become stronger, when you practice release of energetic holding, you feel more at ease and able to positively condition your conscious mind. It is through your intellect (buddhi) that you are able to learn new habits and release old ways of being by directing where your attention goes. Through your meditation practices, you are able to strengthen this aspect of mind while clearing away impressions from the senses and graspings of identity that cloud mind space. As your intellect strengthens, you begin to have more control over the accumulation of the senses and the grasping of ego, allowing mind space to remain clear and calm—another lovely example of the individual aspects working together as a united system toward balance.

Through all of this, you are gradually transforming your conscious mind. While the essence of *chitta* is pure, it becomes clouded by thoughts and grasping of ego. There is a concept known as *chitta suddhi*, which translates as "purification of consciousness" and is considered the very purpose of yoga, that allows us to reconnect to the truth we are beneath the clutter of distraction.[11] Ripples of thought can cause the mind to become chaotic, and it is only when they are still that we can connect to pure consciousness. Through obtaining this purified state of mind, we can realize true self by releasing attachments to ego and ripples of thought waves. To achieve this state, we simply practice all aspects of yoga, especially the eight limbs of practice and teachings of the *Yoga Sutras*.

Chapter 6

Calming the Fluctuations of Mind

Allow your eyes to close and your awareness to turn inward.
Notice the current feeling of you...

Feel the body release any unnecessary holding
and the ease of being that then flows into those spaces.
Feel the expansiveness of your being...
lower body releasing into the earth, crown of the head moving
toward the sky,
space of shoulders softening, subtle lift of the chest, widening of
collarbones,
subtle lift of the chin, lengthening of the neck,
and releasing all the muscles of the face.

Observe the natural movement occurring in your still body...
rhythm of the belly...ribs...chest...stream of effortless breath in and
out of the nose,
the feeling of your body naturally breathing.

Then notice the space behind your eyes and forehead, the space of
your mind.
Feel as if the space of your mind is a pond of water—imagine it
calm, clear, and expansive. Fluctuations will arise through the pull
of the senses or thought stream...
allow these, just as a gentle breeze, to move through and only
subtly affect mind space.
Then return to your open, spacious state.

Yoga is the union of your awareness with all that is. It is yoking
your consciousness to your current experience of living, allowing

you to connect with your true self in each moment and witness life from this view. This experience of connection that the practices of yoga cultivate is a peaceful state of ultimate union and oneness that can best be described as sinking into a state of pure *being*. To attain this deep connection, we simply utilize the practice, yet self-discipline is necessary. It is a commitment to yourself—a dedication to including nourishing thoughts and activities in your day that, in turn, help you feel more balanced and peaceful in each moment of your life. While struggles may arise, as they do with any new habit or routine, setting the goal to move forward each day, step by step, is a way of honoring that which you are in this life. Once you begin to learn the concepts and utilize the practices, you will experience glimpses of your awareness starting to merge with the present moment, and this union will gradually begin to feel more obtainable and sustainable as a state of being. As you continue to calm mind space and connect to this peaceful state, a gradual shift from living in a state of doing to living in a state of being emerges.[1]

Through practice, we calm the "fluctuations of the mind" that occur through living. All of the activity in mind space creates clutter and cloudiness that affect how we experience life. Imagine your space of mind as a pool of clear, calm water—this is its natural state. When the water is transparent and tranquil, you can see the base of the pool and all that is in it clearly; as you witness life through the water, you can view your environment with clarity. Yet thoughts arise that cause subtle waves, old stories and memories create little whirlpools, and emotions cloud the water, making it difficult to witness the world around you and connect inward as it is hard to see. The main purpose of yoga is to quiet and calm the space of mind (chitta) so that it can return to its natural state.[2] A lucid and serene state of mind creates the conditions for you to *rediscover* who you are and always have been beneath the layers of distraction by allowing you a closer view of each aspect of your being within each present moment. It is there that you are able to experience yourself and the world around you distinctly. Through this clarity, you are able to achieve *self-realization*…not creating any sort of new self but rediscovering that which has always been there—the truth of you versus the emotions, thoughts, ideas, triggers, and stories of who you have thought yourself to be, your true nature at the core of your being. Once discovered, there is no need to analyze or try to figure out what your true self is; you are just cleaning up mind space, allowing it to settle, and witnessing the calm, peaceful, pure being of *you* that is revealed.[3]

Your true self is realized as a result of the *stilling of the mind*. When fluctuations and cloudiness are present, you tend to think—*This is me…I **am** these thoughts, emotions, and memories*. You may then identify with these thought patterns and even start to take them on as false identities and behaviors. Think of a time when you were so immersed in negative thoughts about something that they started to consume your focus and then the feelings that arose caused all of your thoughts, even those unrelated to the current situation, to reflect a negative tone. Even your words, emotions, and actions may have emanated this vibe. The calming of your mind is an ongoing process, as the mind is continually attracted to your external environment, which affects the "waters of the mind" through subtle winds and waves. Yet with a baseline of clarity, you can better distinguish what is "you" from what it is that you perceive. There is "you," your true self, the witness of experience, and then there is all that can be witnessed. Once you realize that these shifting winds can affect the mind but cannot change who is witnessing mind space, you are able to maintain that clarity and consciously choose not to take on the identity of thoughts and emotions. When you are not practicing stillness of the mind, the waves and cloudiness can, once again, become the norm, and you can fall back into a pattern of identifying with them. This is why practice is key. The regression into clouded consciousness is subtle enough that you can fall back into previous thought patterns while being completely unaware this has occurred. As you practice releasing your attachments to the chatter of mind and moving into the seat of the observer, you will get better at it. You can then notice when you get wrapped up in emotions and release them before a deeper attachment occurs. It is also much easier to keep something clean when you tend to it every day than when you tend to it only occasionally and have many layers of clutter to work through.[4]

Within the totality of practice, there are two foundational elements that help us learn how to achieve and maintain this calm state of mind: effort and non-attachment. To develop a clear and tranquil mind space through the practices, we must do them. Then we cultivate the ability to release our attachment to outcomes, temptations, and habitual thought processes. The combination of the two helps us navigate life with more balance and a peaceful baseline of being as they continue to positively affect each other. The effort of practice helps us let go of attachments, and this release helps practice seem effortless. The eight limbs of yoga, utilized in a systematic way, allow us to cultivate a calm mind space, and the practice of non-attachment creates clarity. It is a gradual shift toward learning to release and then being able to truly let go.[5]

When we are no longer holding on to past stories or future concerns, we can more skillfully and productively experience life because a calm, spacious mind is a healthy state of mind. In an unhealthy state, the mind feels full and constricted as it grasps and clings to all distractions of environment, thoughts, and emotions. When we create space in mind, our physical and energetic bodies reflect this, allowing us to gradually ungrasp in every layer of our being. It is through our practice that we become aware of the grasping, at a surface level as well as at a deeper level of sensory memories and patterns. This is where we have the opportunity to ungrasp and create space, diving deeper into unconscious attachments that are affecting how we perceive ourselves and our environments.[6] The main elements that affect state of mind are the quality of operating, the clarity within, and all of the mental pathways created by thoughts. These are the aspects that distort your perception and that you are releasing through your practice and through non-attachment. The more deeply you understand what you are working with, the better you become at witnessing the mind and knowing what to release.

Quality of Functioning

The mind functions at varying levels, from barely working to performing optimally as well as a few in between. Similar to how the quality of a car's engine affects all of the moving parts, how well the mind is operating radiates into all aspects of our being. Our meditation practice allows us to enhance the quality of chitta, helping all of the other aspects of mind reach their full potential. When operating at its lowest level, the mind feels agitated and restless. This state is often described as "monkey mind," where our attention swings from branch to branch like a monkey, bouncing off of random thoughts, emotions, and perceptions without any rhyme or reason.[7] In this state of mind, it feels impossible to focus on anything, make a decision, or be present. Operating in this low-functioning mode eventually creates energetic and physical states of anxiety or panic. Moving through your day in this fast-paced, multi-tasking mode can become habitual for your state of mind so that, even when you want to relax or focus on one thing at a time, it feels impossible to do so.

The next level is a bit better but still not ideal. This level is described as creating the feeling of a "heavy water buffalo standing for hours on end in one place."[8] In this state, we feel sluggish and dull in mind with no interest or urge to do much of anything. It is a feeling of deep mental fatigue that radiates throughout our whole being as if our energetic cup is empty. This level of functioning can occur through instances such as eating too much, getting too little sleep, taking certain medications, experiencing grief or deep disappointment, or operating from a chaotic state of "monkey mind" for too long.

In the third level of functioning, the mind has movement, yet there is no consistency, purpose, or direction, as it is easily distracted. Without the ability to focus, the mind has difficulty overcoming obstacles and doubts that arise, causing feelings of uncertainty and lack of confidence to emerge.[9] In this state, we may feel as if we are just going through the motions of life, with oscillating motivation, lethargy, or boredom, rather than truly living. We want to do something, but obstacles distract us. We lose confidence and may even feel incapable of moving forward toward our goals, as if they are out of reach or not within our realm of achieving. Unfortunately, it is thought that this is the most common state of mind.

In the fourth level, the mind is clear and any distractions that come along have little influence. In this state, the mind is able to focus, which gives us the ability to have direction, move toward goals, and continue to keep our attention on them.[10] In this state of mind, we feel as if anything is possible, we are motivated, and we can see the means to accomplishing our objectives. When obstacles of doubt or uncertainty arise, they do not distract us from the task at hand. This is the quality of mind that we are setting as our standard. Then, if we fall into lower-functioning states, we will be able to recognize this with more ease and return to that baseline of operating. Every time we meditate, we turn up the "tuner" of mental functioning so that, with daily practice, we are able to reach and maintain this state as our norm, our baseline for experiencing life. This is achievable because, when our mind enters a meditative state, it is functioning at the fifth level, the highest state at which the mind can operate. At this level of functioning, "the mind is linked completely and exclusively with the object of its attention."[11] Notice this is also the very definition of *meditation*. Here, the mind is functioning in a balanced and stable state, singularly focused and unaffected by external or internal distractions. This is not a mental state we live but one that we find in our practice when in a meditative state. This is why your meditation practice is so important—it allows you to reach your highest level of functioning so that, when you open your eyes and resume your day, you are operating at the "fourth level" in your life.

Clouding of Perception

The clarity of mind is most affected by specific negative mental patterns that cloud *chitta* and distort our perceptions of reality. These misconceptions directly affect how we witness and experience ourselves and our world, as if there were a "filmy layer" covering our view. This concept of that which obscures our view of truth is known as the *kleshas*, which translates as "affliction or poisons" and is thought to be a main source of all human suffering because, when witnessing life through it, we believe that this is our reality.[12] This distorted perception can then affect how we think, act, and feel about what we are experiencing in life. Also known as veils, these obstructions to our view can affect our awareness subtly, perhaps through a tendency of thinking or presuming, or even to the point of blindness to the truth or reality. Because of this, we unnecessarily suffer due to our misconceptions. While we cannot control the physical, mental, or emotional pain we may endure in life, we can control how we perceive and react to it. Just as international Japanese author Haruki Murakami famously states, "Pain is inevitable, suffering is optional."[13]

The first of the five kleshas is known as *avidya*, which translates as "ignorance." The word *vidya* is defined as "correct perception or knowledge" while *a-vidya* means the opposite— "absence of wisdom."[14] When witnessing life through avidya, it is not simply that we lack information; the information is there, but we are unable to see it. This causes an inability to witness the truth about ourselves and others, as we are looking through a clouded lens. It is then, from this view of misperception, that the other four kleshas emerge. One of these is the veil of *asmita*, defined as "egoism, or *I-am*-ness."[15] We all have an aspect of mind known as "ego," yet this obstruction occurs when you identify yourself with the attachments of ego, witnessing life through a self-image that you believe is "who you are," such as *I am worthless* or *I am an angry person*. These thoughts then begin to collect and cover the mind, and you can become trapped within this false narrative. You are none of these things, as all of these thoughts of *what is* are simply shifting occurrences. For example, when you find ourself in a moment of anger or financial struggles, once the emotion subsides or you find a means to more income, these qualities you have claimed are no longer valid. The shifting and changing of your environment and emotions has nothing to do with *who you are* at your core being.

On the other hand, we can also cling to the positive elements of your ego, creating thoughts such as—*I am the best, I am right*, or *Only I know*. This attachment to thoughts centered on "I am" causes you to view life from a clouded perspective focused only on how everything affects you and prevents you from feeling connected to your true self and others around you.

Another obstruction that can arise is known as *raga*, defined as "attachment or desires."[16] This is the distraction or pull of thoughts about things or experiences that bring fleeting moments of satisfaction but do not create lasting joy. It is the desire to have something that was once pleasurable even if it was not helpful for you. These urges cloud the mind with feelings of needing these experiences in order to feel happy, which is how all addictions and unhelpful habits arise. Due to the clouded lens you are looking through, you feel if you cannot acquire this, you will suffer; yet even when you do obtain it, the pleasure fades. As you continue the search for it all over again, a habitual cycle is created.

This veil also affects your life, creating unnecessary suffering and disappointment when aspects of your life do not live up to your attachment to the outcomes you feel you need or desire. This can deceive you into thinking that long-lasting happiness lies outside of you rather than being cultivated from within.

The next obscurity we can begin to cultivate is the opposite of this, as it causes an aversion toward events, people, or situations from the past that have produced unpleasant feelings. It is known as *dvesha* and is described as "repulsion or distaste."[17] In this state, you begin to witness things, people, and experiences through a lens of previous negative feelings that cause you to develop prejudgments, prejudices, or preconceived ideas about certain groups of people or environments. When you are unable to avoid these experiences, or even have to think about encountering them, you suffer through feelings of dread and anxiety. This can also create avoidance and a disconnect from those around you who do not share the same views or ways of "seeing" the world. This obstruction of the mind can even reach a degree where it leads to discrimination and injustices, as it obscures your perspective of reality—we are all one; there is no separation.

The last of the veils is *abhinivesha,* defined as "fear."[18] It tends to be the most subtle, as it slowly accumulates over time. It is also the most common klesha, as it collects through deeply buried past and present experiences or even future worries of things yet to occur. This aspect can seep into all facets of your life through fear of actual things or experiences, the unknown, uncertainty, loss, or simply change. The root of all fear-based thoughts and actions is derived from concerns that something undesirable might happen to you and your life. This is an instinct that is meant to help you survive, yet it can cause you to become fearful when you overestimate risks.

When viewing life through a veil of fear, we suffer by missing out on opportunities to enjoy and connect to the world around us and parts of ourselves unexplored. This causes us to cling to the tangible, physical self as if that is who we are, yet this only causes more suffering as the body inevitably continues to change over time. We can become sick or hurt, and we will grow older. While we cannot stop change from occurring, we do have the ability to choose how we perceive and react to it. A clear view from which to witness life is imperative.

The *kleshas* can affect our view individually and collectively. When we are witnessing life through them, it can be incredibly difficult to understand that what we are observing is not truly reality. Ironically, we are more aware of them in their absence than in their presence. When we see something clearly, we feel a sense of peace inside us without tension, uncertainty, or agitation. It is when the veils lift and clarity arises that we realize the distinction. Also remember that these veils develop gradually over time, making it difficult to witness the shift from reality to misperception; therefore, it takes time to lift them as well. Once we are able to rid the mind of one layer, we may begin to discover deeper layers that exist. One of the primary purposes of all of our yoga practices is to remove these afflictions of the mind that cause eventual suffering. The most helpful practices for overcoming the kleshas are pranayama (yogic breathing), dhyana (meditative state), tapas (self-discipline), and svadhyaya (self-study). Through these practices, we are able to lift the veils, witness more clarity, and become more aware as the gathering of the kleshas occurs.

Whenever we witness life from within this murky view, it is our practice that shines a light through the distortion. We can then be more aware when disillusion starts to cloud the truth. As we continue with practice, we become able to prevent afflictions from accumulating in the first place by utilizing the tools daily to clear up mind space.[19]

Mental Grooves

Every thought, connected with emotion and action, leaves behind a subtle residue known as *samskaras*.[20] These become mental impressions that create imprints that your mind continues to revisit. Every time one of these thought streams is revisited, emotions are felt, and an action is performed, it deepens mental grooves that begin to create stronger thought patterns, eventually leading to deep-seated habits that greatly influence how you move through and perceive your life. For example, think of a time when you felt "triggered," like someone was "pushing your buttons." In a moment like this, the mind instantly goes down a mental pathway that brings up old stories about similar situations that have occurred in the past.

As soon as the mind encounters these memories, you immediately feel the emotions of those previous moments, which creates mental and—at times—physical reactions that can govern your perceptions of the current situation and our response to it. Often, we are unaware that our current thought patterns are being dictated by old emotions and past memories. Instead, we feel and experience them as if they are valid and completely relevant to the present moment. Similar to a worn path in a field well-traveled over time, these deep mental grooves become more difficult to avoid as they develop into addictions and habitual modes of being.

The importance of being conscious of this process is that, if you are not aware of falling into old pathways and patterns, these stories will continue to play out in the background of your mind. The previous dialogues and stories you have become accustomed to telling yourself will start to mold your perception, govern your choices, become patterns, and eventually become ways of *being*. For example, imagine that, as a child, you were around large erratic dogs that deeply frightened you and this experience molded your view of dogs in general. In your early adult life, if you saw a dog, you became filled with anxiety and fear, feeling as if every dog could not be trusted and may hurt you. Then you stopped spending time with friends who had dogs and going to places where dogs might be encountered. Yet this was just a perception of reality clouded by previous thoughts and emotions that molded your view. In reality, while some dogs can have dangerous tendencies, they are generally sweet, loving, wonderful companions. Once you stop revisiting this story, it will become quieter and eventually stop being something you hold on to at all as you start to have new experiences with dogs, interacting with some that are kind, trustworthy, and friendly. This scenario exemplifies how thoughts or dialogues based on your experiences can lead to ways of perceiving the world around you even though the only place they truly exist is in your mind. These perceptions are not "you," as they too can shift and change.

We become most aware of these mental grooves in meditation. Through our journey of practice, once we release our mental grasping of body, energetic holding, and outward distractions, we enter mind space. Then we can observe the chatter of thoughts that reside there that usually go unnoticed as we spend most of our lives distracted. As we connect to this space, we are also able to witness the mind falling through or riding streams of thoughts that stem from outward distractions. For instance, you hear a firetruck and a thought stream is triggered—*I wonder where it's going...I hope everyone is okay...The other day I heard an ambulance...I've been hearing a lot of sirens lately*...and so on. Or you smell some food cooking—*I wonder what that is...It smells delicious...I'm kind of hungry...What will I have for dinner?...I should go to the store*...and so on. When we encounter these distractions of thought in mind space, our tendency is to grasp and ride those streams of thought. All of this chatter in mind space does not appear because you are meditating; it was already there, in the background, influencing your perception of each new moment. Your practice is not only where you become aware of the chatter but also the means to gradually release it. This is the dual

95

purpose of the practice: strengthening focus by releasing grasping and clearing away the unnecessary clutter you discover. As you improve your ability to shift your focus away from deep mental grooves, you stop reinforcing old patterns and the old dialogue begins to dissipate and fade away, as it is no longer applicable to your current reality. You then awaken to a healthier state of being where you can see the truth of each moment through strong focus and clarity.

Discover ~ Release ~ Replenish

The samskaras of the mind eventually affect all aspects of our being—emotional, energetic, and physical. When your mind travels down an old stream of thought that triggers a previous emotional response, this can create a rush of anxiety through the body, physical tension may arise, and breath may become shallow. This is just one of a myriad of ways that samskaras can affect each layer of your being. Thankfully, your practice allows you to connect to each layer, releasing old patterns that are unhelpful while, at the same time, creating new supportive and open ways of being. From the first moment of practice, you connect to the current feeling of your body, noticing tension or holding, and then move toward softening and strengthening. You continue with this method of discovery, release, and replenishment in your pranic body, senses, and focus as you utilize each exploratory tool of the eight limbs, enabling you to connect and move through each layer. As you release old negative samskaras, the practices themselves create new positive ways of being. These new thoughts and emotions create beneficial impressions in mind, prana, and body that activate positive habits, routines, and ways of feeling. For example, your asana practice helps you discover habitual holding patterns in the body, release them, and create new ways of posture. This is also true in your pranic body as you clear energetic blocks or stagnation through pranayama. Being able to release the old and unhelpful patterns in your body and energy is key, as how you *feel* in your body greatly affects your perception, thought process, and understanding of life—not only how you witness life but also how you move, think, and act within it.

As you weaken the pull toward these distractions, you also reduce their effects and your mind space returns to its natural state, as pure as a pond of crystal clear water, allowing you to easily see all within. In this calm mind, you can more clearly witness deep habits and thought patterns and release underlying samskaras that may be unconsciously affecting you. With this clear view that is free of distractions, you gain the ability to focus and be truly present in both the smallest and biggest moments of your life. As like attracts like, in this state, the mind is more attracted to that which is positive, joyous, or nurturing and turns away from that which is negative, painful, or destructive. When you are feeling calm and peaceful, everything around you is witnessed through this light and reflects the beauty that you radiate from within. Our perspective completely alters our reality. With a tranquil and clear state of mind, our world becomes a little brighter as well. The more consistently we are able to live in this state of being, the more we will attract healthful energy into our lives. Often referred to as "living yoga," the practice is not only utilizing the techniques to create this state of being but is also living in this new mode of being and how it positively affects our self-perception and our ability to attract a more peaceful baseline from which to experience life.[21]

This healthy, spacious state of mind, energy, and body is known as *sukha*, translated as "good space."[22] Our practice helps us to obtain and maintain living in a state of sukha. This is a sense of ease throughout our being; more than a surge of emotions such as joy or happiness, it is a deep lasting feeling of comfort within. The opposite of this state is known as *duhkha*, defined as "bad space." This is the encompassing feeling of discomfort, suffering, or being stuck and restricted in the mind and in life.[23] In this state,

97

we may feel like our goals are completely out of reach or we have no means to overcome obstacles. This can seep into the bigger dreams we have as well as the seemingly insignificant decisions and situations that take place in our lives. When we are living in a state of sukha, we feel light and open in our whole being as if anything is possible and there are no limits to the goodness we are available to and can create in our lives.

We unconsciously create and collect feelings of duhkha through our actions, responses, or decisions that arise from incorrect perceptions due to cloudiness of the mind. This is why the kleshas are thought to be the main source of suffering—when witnessing life through them, we begin to cultivate a feeling of "bad space." Imagine wanting a new job that requires training to apply and having to witness this experience through old veils of misperception and negative thoughts, such as—*School was difficult before, so I don't want to bother with it again* (aversion), *I am not a good student...I am not an academic* person (egoism), *I probably won't get it anyway...even if I did get the job, it might not work out* (fear)...*It's not a good job anyway, and I would never be able to achieve it* (ignorance). Then, because of all of these incorrect perceptions from witnessing this situation inaccurately through the veils (kleshas), you decide not to pursue the job at all. Later, you start to feel stuck in your current job, as if you have no ability to move ahead and gain financial stability or fulfillment. Ultimately, you feel mentally restricted by the distractions of obstacles that seem like boundaries you are unable to overcome (duhkha). This sequence of actions resulting from misconception, creates a variety of suffering, especially if it becomes a common occurrence over time. All aspects of our yoga practice help us release feelings of duhkha by cultivating "good space" (sukha) within. The practices also allow us to lift the veils of misperception, eliminating the collection of duhkha in the first place.

Living Yoga

Once you start practicing and embodying the benefits that arise, you naturally begin to live more united, connected, and present in each moment. Once you start creating a peaceful and balanced state of being, every moment can be an opportunity to cultivate more of this in your life, as you will continue to attract more good simply by living in this calm, positive state. You can also bring your conscious awareness to implementing the practices in your day, such as utilizing the yamas in each interaction with your environment and the niyamas in caring for yourself. Through asana practice on the mat, you cultivate the ability to consciously bring your physical body into a balanced state of stability and ease at any time and allow your pranic body to be open and freely flowing. With your mind able to focus and release distractions through your meditation practice, you can operate and experience life in a clear, calm light and abide in "good space." In this state of being, a greater clarity arises as you experience a more connected way of being.

When you are in tune with your body and something feels off, you can detect the source of the problem and identify a solution more easily. Similarly, the mind benefits when you are able to live in a more calm and clear mental state. Your practice helps you find clarity and, through this, your mind space gains greater illumination for witnessing all of the workings of chitta. When you are able to view your own mind clearly, your practice becomes more than just a way to maintain this state—it is also a means to witnessing deeper levels of consciousness and the seeds of profound mental grooves, enabling you to release and clear them. Your practice then becomes that which clears mind space as well as a tool for obtaining knowledge from what is discovered. Once noticed, you can then nourish or release whatever is revealed. This becomes one of the most beneficial aspects of your journey within.[24]

This process also allows you to develop the ability to connect to your own insight and wisdom in all of your daily moments. For once, the mental chatter begins to quiet and clear awareness arises. Insights you may never have noticed before can be witnessed and understood. By releasing the old mental clutter, stories, and dialogues that were previously occupying the mind, you create space for inner wisdom to flood in. Through practice, these moments become more frequent and, eventually, you are able to live in a state of open awareness *most of the time*. Then, when you are feeling not so clear, you can come back to the cushion and reconnect with that inner knowing and truth.

Chapter 7

Guidebook to Caring for Self

Notice what it feels like to pause all doing or trying and just be...
awareness resting on the current feeling of your body,
feeling of your body breathing,
feeling of the current space of your mind.

At that point of stillness, allow your awareness to gently expand...
exploring the areas of natural movement in body,
the textures and sensations of the environment on your skin,
the temperature of the air, subtle sounds around you...
no grasping or searching, just gentle expansion of effortless
awareness.

Continuing with this feeling of open, limitless being,
draw your awareness back inward to the feeling of you...
easeful being, spacious state of mind, natural rhythm of breath...
sink into the natural effortless feeling of YOU be-ing.

The movement of life leads us toward the extremes of excessive and depleted states of being. To care for yourself within this flow of continuous change, the key is to consciously guide yourself toward balance. Change itself does not have a positive or negative quality, which allows you to choose which quality you bring in. You can utilize mindful, positive daily choices to continually guide yourself back to center. It is an ongoing process of sinking into mindful *being*, in whatever you may be doing, with the only destination being each "now moment," as Eric Schiffman would say. This is the foundational benefit of yoga: experiencing moments of clarity and connection in your body, breath, and mind and becoming able to emulate that peaceful union within each moment of your life. This ability to extend your experience from practice into your life occurs subtly at first, gradually radiating into your whole mode of being with steady practice. T.K.V. Desikachar describes, "In yoga we are simply trying to create the conditions in which the mind becomes as useful as possibly for our actions. This can only happen gradually—every shortcut is an illusion. It is a step-by-step process, one that includes a great number of techniques from which one must choose intelligently according to the individual need. The *Yoga Sutras* give many suggestions, which together comprise our yoga practice, the yoga sadhana."[1]

Rather than another task for your to-do list, your yoga practices are the foundational support that helps you move through all of your daily experiences with more ease and focus. You can start your day without eating, drinking water, or exercising and still function, yet not optimally. If you eat, you will feel more nourished. If you drink, you will feel more hydrated. If you move your body, you will feel more energetic and stable. And if you meditate, you will feel more clear and peaceful. Meditating is not only beneficial for some; it is science available to all. We are all stronger than our deepest habits. The core of your being is inherently calm and peaceful; you just have to weed through distractions and bad habits in order to find it. Then, through practice, you stay connected to it. It is the small steps continued daily that will make the biggest changes in your life.

All of our yoga practices create a pure, peaceful quality known as *sattva* in the body, energy, and mind.[2] In contrast to very busy or sedentary activities that cultivate those same qualities within us, we can embody a state of emotional, mental, and physical equilibrium through practicing activities that are harmonious and balanced. This is best understood by starting at the beginning of yoga philosophy in which there are two fundamental principles of the nature of existence known as *purusha* and *prakriti*. Your soul, pure consciousness, the seer of experience, the witness of life, is *purusha*. Everything else in the everchanging nature of our reality is known as *prakriti*.[3] This includes the environment, the body, energy, and mind—all of the things that can be observed and witnessed by purusha (your unchanging soul). Everything in nature is continually shifting. All of the aspects of living that you can observe can and will change. The environment around you continues to move through seasons in which you grow, you age, and your energy and thoughts fluctuate. While this change happens naturally, it is also your means of transformation. Rolf Sovik, president and spiritual director of the Himalayan Institute, describes, "Prakriti is a reservoir of limitless potential consisting of three fundamental forces."[4] By understanding these forces of nature, you can learn how to shift the quality of your whole being in a positive direction toward peace and balance.

Qualities of Nature

The three fundamental forces of prakriti are known as the *gunas*. These are *sattva* (purity and balance), *rajas* (movement and drive), and *tamas* (stillness and darkness).[5] All three qualities are always present within us and within all of nature at varying levels. Through your choices and interactions with nature, you have the ability to intentionally alter these levels in your body and mind. Through your daily activities and moments, you can consciously "cultivate sattva and reduce raja and tamas to a working minimum."[6] We need an abundance of sattva to elevate our state of peace and harmony. We want enough rajasic quality for drive and passion but not so much that we feel anxiousness and longing. We need enough tamas for stability and rest but not too much, which causes lethargy and dullness. Each quality within you can be elevated or reduced through your interactions with external objects and your lifestyle, activities, behaviors, practices, and thoughts. This concept is similar to the phrase "You are what you eat" but with a broader application, referencing not only the food you digest but everything you take in and consume from your environment. Once you understand how the gunas operate and affect your state of being, you can understand the "feel" of each guna and use that knowledge as a guide to move toward a more sattvic state of being.

The gunas affect us through everything we take in and digest—this includes food, energy, emotions, experiences, and thoughts. Reducing the amount of tamasic and rajasic qualities that we take in and infusing more nourishing qualities of sattva into our daily meals and activities helps us gradually move toward a *sattvic state of living*. The quality of tamas in nature is heavy and dense. A little of this quality is helpful for creating stability and groundedness, yet too much causes dullness and cloudiness in mind. Tamasic foods are lifeless, processed, stale, or impure, such as heavy meats, leftovers, and chemically treated ingredients. Tamasic activities are passive, sedentary, dull, and mindless, such as oversleeping, overeating, and performing monotonous tasks. Too much tamasic quality within can lead to a lack of energy and enthusiasm, procrastination, and blindness to reality and our personal truths. Rajas, on the other hand, is the quality of energy, action, change, and movement. It is the force behind passion, desire, and effort although, in excess, it creates a quality of unsteadiness, agitation, and unhappiness that manifests in the mind and strengthens the pull of our attachments. This longing for some sort of stability within the chaos causes us to grasp on to outcomes and the comfort of previous habits, even if they are detrimental to us. Rajasic activities include overexercising, overworking, excessive thinking, or habitually operating in a mode of busyness in mind and body. This creates feelings of anxiety and racing thoughts, as if we "cannot sit still." There is also an excess of this quality in foods that are fried or contain stimulants or intense spice. Consuming these in moderation and with awareness of how they affect us is key.

The quality of sattva is the energy of purity, harmony, and balance. Cultivating more sattva in our lives not only creates more of these attributes within us but also helps us reduce qualities of excess rajas and tamas. Activities that increase sattva are those that create joy and positive thoughts as well as all yogic practices, which were developed to create sattva in mind and body. In general, sattvic foods are whole grains, legumes, and fresh fruits and vegetables, yet it is important to understand that the gunas do not describe an *object* but rather the current *quality of the object*. For example, if you pick a ripe apple off of a tree, at that time, it is full of sattvic quality. If you eat it, you will then feel the nourishing sattvic quality within. Pick the same apple but, instead, cut it up, cover it in a sweet batter, and fry it. The apple will then be predominant in rajasic quality, and if you consume it, you will take on this same quality. Take that fried apple and put the leftover pieces in the refrigerator, then eat them the next day. The apple would then be predominant in tamasic quality and eating it would create that same feeling within. This principle applies to our activities as well. You can go for a walk on a busy street or with racing thoughts and have a very rajasic experience. You can also go for a walk on a beautiful day at the beach with no one around while your mind is focused on the peaceful surroundings and have a very sattvic experience. Alternatively, you could be inching forward in a slow-moving line, having a very tamasic experience while feeling a lethargic, dull, and mindless quality within.

Every day, we move our bodies, breathe, and think. Our yoga practices embody these same activities but with the added quality of *sattva*. In fact, all of our yoga techniques and tools were developed to create a harmonious and united quality in the mind and body. Each individual technique in the totality of living yoga possesses the qualities of purity, peace, and balance. Through our practice, we gradually shape our overall sense of being and experience of living into a more sattvic state. The first step is to understand that your interactions with the gunas (qualities of nature) are always occurring and subtly affecting you, most of the time outside of your conscious awareness. Yet once you are able to notice and observe the qualities of the natural world, you start to recognize the way each feels and can detect these distinctive qualities in your diet, thoughts, habits, and activities. Imagine walking down a busy city street (rajas) versus a quiet walk in the woods (sattva). Imagine the feeling of being on a deadline at work with only minutes to spare (rajas) versus a relaxing soak in a lavender bath (sattva). Reflect on the feeling of a wonderful evening connecting and laughing with friends (sattva) versus a night of lying on the couch mindlessly scrolling through your phone (tamas). In imagining all of these scenarios, you can remember how those activities directly impact the quality of your *feeling of being*.

Another large component of that which we take in is food. You can connect to how you *feel* after consuming a fresh piece of fruit (sattva) versus a large cup of coffee (rajas) or a leftover piece of food (tamas). Through your diet and your sensory perceptions, you consume and digest all of the qualities of your environment, activities, behaviors, and food. Once you notice how these elements create these same attributes within you, you can begin to bring more balanced, harmonious qualities into your life through your behaviors and choices. If you are feeling imbalanced, you now know what to adjust in order to move toward a more balanced state. Through this discovery, you also become more aware of your own tendencies toward specific actions that may be creating imbalances, such as desiring caffeine in the afternoon or becoming a couch potato after overeating at dinnertime. In addition, you become better at recognizing the intuitive choices you have been making all along that help bring you into balance, such as enjoying a daily walk in nature or taking deep, full breaths after a stressful moment. Once you are able to witness, observe, and understand the qualities in your environment as well as your unconscious habits, you can begin to cultivate a deeper sense of peace and well-being in all aspects of your life through sattvic choices, behaviors, and attitudes.

Hills, Valleys, and Quicksand

Throughout life, there will be highs, lows, and even times when we feel so immersed in a current circumstance or state that we feel stuck or unable to get beyond it. While each of our specific circumstances and feelings are completely valid and personal, it is important to be able to step back and see the "big picture" in order to realize these are all simple occurrences of the human condition. Thousands of years ago, ancient humans were encountering these same barriers in life, so much so that they discovered how to overcome them. The ups and downs of the human experience are just obstacles that arise along the path of living. The journey toward ease in body and clarity of mind is not linear. We will have moments of great elation and peace as well as experiences completely lacking these blissful qualities. Once we are able to recognize these obstacles that arise as simply something to overcome rather than something that prevents us from moving forward, the ebb and flow of life will no longer hold us back from living in a state of balance, clarity, and well-being. Our practice helps us with this.

There are certain obstacles known as *antarayas* that can occur within and cause us to fall out of practice. Desikachar describes how the *Yoga Sutras* presents this concept as "...rocks lying on the path traveled by someone who has set off on the yoga journey. The student is constantly stumbling over them, making detours, or getting stuck."[7] The antarayas are depicted in both yoga philosophy and Buddhist teachings as hurdles, stumbling blocks, and obstructions along the path toward mental and physical enlightenment, health, and well-being. They can each arise on their own, yet they also cause others to emerge. There are nine specific obstacles that can cause us to fall out of practice. These are not just thoughts or moments that make us lose motivation for our practice but encompassing feelings of being that seem like a barrier to practicing, so much so that we may give up or stop for extended periods of time. This concept is not unique only to the practice of yoga and meditation; it can be applied to any activity we are practicing or infusing into our life for the betterment of our well-being, including eating well, exercising, learning, and so on.

One of these obstacles is *illness*. When you are sick, hurt, or do not feel well, it directly affects the state of your mind. Unable to move freely due to pain or enduring other physical ailments is a mentally consuming process. At first, this focus on healing is a necessary function. Yet, over time, if you do not allow your awareness to release the distraction of the body, it can cause your mind to feel out of balance and you can fall out of practice. Another obstacle that may arise is *lethargy*. This is more than just being tired or having feelings of physical fatigue; this is a feeling of low energetic drive or passion, a lack of enthusiasm that can create a feeling of mental dullness and sluggish focus. Lethargy can also lead to the next obstacle of *doubt*, which is typically considered one of the most common to arise as we start to progress in our yoga practices. You may begin to feel as if you cannot keep up with your practice, that it is not for you, that it is not really helping, or that it is not really worth it.

Feelings of *impatience* can also present themselves when you do not progress quickly enough or when you take steps backwards instead of forwards. You may have times in your life when your responsibilities and experiences create *fatigue* through physical and mental exhaustion. When life gets especially busy, whether it be related to the holidays, your job, your family, or other life circumstances that cause *distraction*, your practice can fall off schedule. *Arrogance* can also create barriers to moving forward, as you may think you already know everything. And the opposite can be true when you feel *overwhelmed* by continuing to move forward in practice to the extent of feeling incapable of taking a new step, even when it would benefit you. In turn, this can cause *a loss of confidence,* as you may feel that caring for yourself in this way is not important or that you are not worth it. These

108

thoughts and feelings can even begin to manifest as a negative attitude, physical suffering, or cloudiness in mind. While each of these obstacles can feel like a road block on our journey inward, it is our commitment to *practice* that allows us to overcome them.

Cultivating a Sadhana

The philosophies and practices of yoga, especially the eight limbs, help us overcome and remove barriers along the journey of life by creating more ease and clarity. While the tendency is to allow obstacles that arise to stop you from practicing, it is the *practice* that will actually eliminate them. Once you become aware of them, you can more easily detect when they start to appear or are present within you. This simple awareness helps you to witness the barrier for what it is so you can mentally step outside of the intensity of an encompassing experience of illness, impatience, fatigue, or loss of confidence and into the viewpoint of an observer. By doing this, you can experience it as the transcendent, fleeting, and fluctuating moment it is as opposed to a solid, tangible obstacle in your permanent reality. As you continue with your practice, caring for self, you can prevent your current feeling from derailing you too far from a balanced state. Without sinking in and grasping on to the feeling, allowing it to distract you from doing what helps you *feel good*, these barriers will gradually lift and move out of your way. This concept of a routine daily practice is known as *sadhana*, which is a Sanskrit term describing more than just a new habit to feel better in this moment or an occasional activity that may eventually get us to a desired state; it is a disciplined method of practice for accomplishing a specific goal.[8] A "sadhana practice" is not a specific technique but rather describes a practitioner's consistent use of tools on a daily basis with the goal of connecting to true Self and present moment. The teachings and practices of yoga—particularly the eight limbs—support our sadhana by aiding us in the release of our attachments to ego so as to achieve union with mind, body, soul, and all that is.

Intention Matters

We can learn about something, and possibly even experience it, yet for it to truly help us, we must put it into action. It is when we start to apply the knowledge that we begin to cultivate the benefits. The spectrum of a yoga practice is broad and expansive, so the foundational intention and energy that we bring into play is of the utmost importance, especially when using them in our daily sadhana. Bringing our yoga into action is known as *kriya*, translated as "to do" or "an action to complete a result."[9] The second chapter of the *Yoga Sutras* reveals three specific types of kriya recommended to achieve the goal of our sadhana. Instead of new techniques or tools, these are simply elements to infuse into our practice, subtle shifts in the underlying purpose of purifying body and mind, learning about Self, and surrendering to all that is. These three components are also subcategories of the niyamas, revealing—once again—the importance of embedding care of self into the action of practice.

The first component is tapas. Not to be confused with external heat therapies for the body, tapas helps create an internal heat to "burn off" physical and mental impurities from within, removing physical toxins, energy blockages, mental attachments, and anything obstructing or clouding our true, pure state of being.[10] This internal fire element is known as *agni* and is our ability to digest and transform everything we take in from our environments including food, thoughts, emotions, sensory elements, and experiences.[11] We can cultivate a strong inner fire through subtle shifts in our practice of the eight limbs. For example, when you infuse your physical posture with ujjayi pranayama and link this breath with repetition of movement such as active twists, laterals, or flexion flow, you are able to create a subtle heat within. There are also specific pranayama techniques that stimulate digestive fire, such as *kapalabhati* (also known as skull shining breath),[12] described in detail in Chapter 7. Another way to bring tapas into your daily routine is by infusing passion, drive, and self-discipline into your life. This is accomplished through learning new things, working toward goals that bring joy, and expanding beyond your comfort zone or what you may have previously felt was out of reach. Both of these aspects help us eliminate unhealthy patterns while, at the same time, creating new positive routines. Small consistent steps over time create the most transformation, and—as with all elements of our practice—balance is key. It is important to approach tapas practice with intention and purpose so that we are able to move into the next foundational element of practice (self-study) with ease.[13]

Once the body, prana, and mind are clear of impurities, you are able to witness more and more of the true self beneath the clutter and distraction. As you begin to submerge into a deeper sense of self, you can more easily move into the next step of kriya known as *svadhyaya* and defined as "to study one's own self."[14] It is a simple shift of observing and learning about yourself while growing in your current practice and life. From the moment you begin your practice and turn your awareness inward, you discover mental chatter and habits of distraction that you may not have been consciously aware of. You may even witness imbalance in how you hold your body, creating underlying aches or tension that can be difficult to detect until misalignment over time causes noticeable pain. Throughout the entire process of utilizing the eight limbs, you are given the opportunity to observe yourself in this deep way. It is then that you can begin to discard the clutter you encounter, learn more about your true self that lies beneath it, and grow in your practice and in life. In your yoga practices, you are not only given a front-row seat to your current state but also a method to witness, discover, and understand it. Then, through tapas, you can cleanse and positively transform this current state and your baseline of being. The more impurities you release, the more of your true self is revealed. For instance, think of your physical body and asana practice—it begins with observing the feeling of body and breath (self-study) and then consciously deepening and lengthening breath through movement (tapas). Throughout the movement and breathwork, you may notice weakness, tension, and tightness or strength, openness, and vitality (self-study). As your routine of the practice (tapas) develops, you start to learn more about your body, see changes and progression, and understand what your body needs. As you clear out physical impurities and misperceptions, you move toward positive transformation (self-study and tapas). The interplay of these two intentional elements applies to all of the limbs of practice.[15]

You can also bring these elements into your life by studying spiritual texts, such as the *Yoga Sutras*. The intention is a bit different than reading other forms of literature, as the information obtained helps you discover more about yourself. When reading these texts, consider how they relate to you, your practice, and your life. In this way, learning infused with svadhyaya will allow you to more deeply explore, reflect, and understand yourself. Another way of practice is simple, mindful awareness of your current moment, being fully present in whatever you are doing and observing all elements of your experience. You can discover so much about yourself, your habits, and areas in need of more balance by witnessing the moments of your life.[16]

The last element recommended to bring into your practice is surrender, also known as *isvara pranidhana*. More specifically translated as "surrendering to the divine,"[17] it helps you loosen your grip on the need to control and place *trust* in a higher divine force beyond your individual body, mind, and singular consciousness. Through this, you put down all of the pressure and weight you are carrying and have confidence that there is something bigger than us occurring. This concept does not imply that you give up. In fact, you are able to apply even more of your focus and effort to the task at hand but in an enjoyable, gentle way. It also does not mean you stop caring. You can care even more deeply when an experience is free of stress and tension, as you can still put forth your best effort without the weight of "clinging" to the details of the outcome. We have limited control over the present moment, the past is already complete, and the future will always be just out of reach. Once we reach the future, it will become the present, where everything we have worked toward in previous present moments has helped us arrive. While we have the ability to create an inner world of clarity and make positive daily choices that move us toward peaceful living and accomplishing our dreams, the exact path, surrounding details, and specific outcomes are yet to be determined. When we consciously relinquish our attachments from our actions to the universal energy that we are a part of, we become lighter and freer and let go of the struggle to control the future unknowns.[18]

It can be difficult to release the notion that we are in control even though our continual grasping of the everchanging world and future outcomes creates only obstacles and eventual suffering in our lives. By infusing the concept of isvara pranidhana into your practice, you cultivate the ability to surrender with more ease in your life, allowing you to physically, energetically, and mentally loosen your grasp on outcomes and place your focus, instead, on the quality of each step along your path. Through asana, you learn how to soften unnecessary tension in the physical body and move through postures where you create strength yet release struggle in order to find ease within stability. Through meditation, you develop the ability to release all of the doing and simply observe natural breath and the workings of the mind. Within this, you discover how to truly listen to yourself, letting go of the need to constantly be doing and choosing a more restful practice instead. This concept of surrendering can continue to ripple out into your daily life by releasing attachments to ego, to the fruits of your actions, to worries, to fears, and—most importantly—by giving up the "illusion of control." As an inner calm develops, you will be able to cultivate a deeper understanding of where genuine, lasting joy and happiness reside, as they have no true tie to outcomes or your self-worth. You will then be able to unlock the hidden capacities of clarity and peace that we all possess underneath the thickening clouds of misperception. Remember that your practice is not about attaining something new; it is simply a way to uncover what is already there, a method for discovering the limitless possibilities that naturally lie deep within you.[19]

Within this process of moving through the koshas with the eight limbs of yoga practices infused with discipline, self-study, and surrender, you can design a practice that is specific to your needs, allowing it to meet you where you are and give you the tools and guidance to return to balance and clarity. For an outline of step-by-step details, see the appendix.

Expanding Asana

While the practice of asana is vast, there are three main methods of utilizing posture for a specific outcome and benefit. We can practice asana in ways beyond just helping our bodies to release daily surface tension and misalignment. It can also help us achieve strength, deep release, and balanced rest. All active asana stems from classical *Hatha Yoga,* dating back to the fourteenth century, with the purpose of preparing us for deep meditation and easeful living through a balanced connection between asana, pranayama, mantra, and mudra. *Ha* is translated as "moon," *tha* as "sun," and *yoga* as "to unite," thus offering techniques to actively *balance the sun and moon energies of the body.*[20] Within this application of asana practice, there is an emphasis on holding postures for a period of time to allow for stretching and strengthening of the muscles along with proper alignment to prevent injuries. When we look at its relationship to Raja Yoga, the eight limbs are the path, and Hatha Yoga provides the method. *The Spirit and Practice of*

Moving into Stillness by Erich Schiffmann is recommended for further study on this topic.

Our yoga practices that have a *yang* energy help us activate the strength and release of our muscles while our practices that have a *yin* energy allow us to target the fascia—the layer of connective tissue that surrounds all of the muscles, joints, and organs in our body. Through Yin Yoga, we utilize seated, prone, and supine postures where we can completely release any doing or activation of the muscles. This allows for a gentle release of the connective tissue surrounding muscle and bones. Fascia is a different substance than muscle, as it has a consistency similar to taffy. If fascia is not worked, it can become dry and brittle, preventing us from moving freely, yet it will become supple and mobile again if we start to slowly work it. To be able to effectively release it, however, we must completely let go of any engagement or doing in the muscle through long, slow holds, gently creating more supple and rehydrated tissue.

The first to introduce this practice in North America was Paulie Zink, martial arts champion who, in the late 1970s, began to fuse the principles of Hatha Yoga with Taoist Yoga in his practice and then taught it to his students. One named Paul Grilley began to study further and teach a fusion of the Yin poses he had learned from Zink with Hatha Yoga, anatomy, and his understanding of the meridians in Chinese acupuncture as well as their relationship to fascia. Subsequently, one of Grilley's students named Sarah Powers began to study and teach the practice while incorporating Buddhist psychology and creating various series of Yin poses to specifically target the meridian systems for health and enlightenment.[21] Recommended reading for further study on this topic is *Yin Yoga: Principles & Practice* by Paul Grilley and *Insight Yoga* by Sarah Powers.

Restorative Yoga is a practice using props to support the body in passive poses that promote deep relaxation and release the effects of stress on the body. This style of yoga was first taught by

B.K.S. Iyengar, a prominent yoga teacher from Bellur, India, who developed a system of poses supported by props to assist the body in healing. The practice was further refined and shared by his student Judith Hanson Lasater who began teaching in the 1970s and spread its application extensively.[22] The practice offers postures designed to move your spine in all directions as every curve of the body is completely supported by blankets, bolsters, and blocks (while in seated, supine, or prone postures) and enjoyed for five to twenty minutes. In these poses, our muscles release tension, also allowing for a subtle release in fascia, yet the primary goals and benefits are deep relaxation, healing, and rejuvenation through activating the parasympathetic nervous system. This aspect of the physical body allows us to "rest and digest" and helps us counter the effects of stress while fortifying our basic functions. *Relax & Renew: Restful Yoga for Stressful Times* by Judith Lasater is recommended for further study on this topic.

Expanding Pranayama

In addition to the pranayama techniques discussed in chapter two, there are also deeper benefits of that practice as well as tools for specific focus. Breathwork helps our physical body by infusing it with oxygen and allowing us to clear and release toxins. Pranayama practices calm and rejuvenate the nervous system while reducing stress and anxiety. They also help reduce avidya, cloudiness of the mind, and reduce *apana* to allow for more prana to flow within. *Apana* is a term that refers to both the force (vayu) of all of the lower body activities of elimination and "rubbish" (a byproduct of undigested food and emotions) that collects when prana is not in balance.[23] Our pranayama techniques help us reduce the apana within through complete exhales, which allow for more prana to flood in through our deep, full inhales. Yoga philosophy describes this concept of the flow of prana:

If a farmer wants to water his terraced fields, he does not have to carry the water in buckets to the various parts of his fields; he has only to open the retaining wall at the top. If he has laid out his terraces well and nothing blocks the flow of the water, it will be able to reach the last field and the furthest blade of grass without help from the farmer. In pranayama we work with the breath to remove blockages in the body. The prana, following the breath, flows by itself into the cleared spaces. In this way we use the breath to make possible the flow of prana.[24]

While all of our yogic breathwork practices help us balance this energy within, there are some that have a more specific focus in order to cultivate a particular benefit.

~ Single Nostril Breath ~

This exercise is similar to nadi shodhana but focused on clearing one pathway versus both. The same hand positioning and method used for alternate nostril breath is used here but following only one path with the inhale continuing in one side and the exhale continuing out the other. This practice is known as *surya bhedana* when inhaling through the right nostril and *chandra bhedana* when inhaling through the left. *Surya (soor-yah)*, translated as "sun," invigorates the body and mind with the warming qualities of the sun and can give us a boost of vitality as it stimulates the nervous system and reduces feelings of sluggishness.[25] *Chandra (chahn-drah)*, translated as "moon," helps us cultivate the calming and cooling qualities of the moon by soothing the nervous system, reducing heat, and allowing us to create a sense of inner balance. *Bhedana (beh-DAH-na)* is defined as "piercing or penetrating," describing how the practice allows us to infuse the mind and body with the energy of the sun or moon.[26]

Bring your pointer finger and middle finger to your third-eye point, center of the forehead, in between the eyebrows. Closing off one side (right or left), take a big deep inhale through the other side. Then close it off and exhale completely through the opposite nostril. Continue repeating in the same direction of flow.

~ Cooling Breath ~

Known as *sitali*, this technique utilizes the sides of the tongue curled up and the peak of the lips while the breath is inhaled slowly through this straw-like shape and then exhaled through the nose.[27] The cooling temperature of the inhale spreads throughout the body, helping to reduce the effects of heat from the environment or inner heat, such as anger or inflammation.

~ Segmented Breath ~

A few forms of pranayama utilize the technique of interrupting the flow of breath, known as *viloma* and translated as "against the natural flow."[28] To energize the body and mind, breathe through the nose, dividing the inhale into segments of four sips of breath followed by one long complete exhale. To bring in more calming and grounding energy, divide the exhale into four segments as if exhaling through a tube as someone pinches it to interrupt your flow. Follow this with a full, complete inhale.

~ Humming (Bee) Breath ~

Known as *bhramari*, this technique uses sound, vibration, and breath to calm the mind and nervous system and directs our focus inward.[29] This technique is incredibly beneficial if you are feeling anxious, unsettled, angry, or irritable, as it helps to open and soften the areas of energy in the heart and throat. To do this, take a deep, full inhale through the nose and then—on each full complete exhale through the nose—add a deep "mmmmmm" sound, as if tasting something surprisingly delicious.

~ Skull Shining Breath ~

Known as *kapalabhati* (*kapala* meaning "skull" and *bhati* meaning "light") this is a technique that emphasizes the exhale through strong, fast abdominal contractions and then allows complete release of doing in order for the inhale to naturally flow in.[30] This contraction in the physical body is subtle and is the same natural effect that occurs as we say a forceful, "Ha!". Give it a try…can you feel it? Now create that same pump of the upper abdomen while exhaling through the nose and making no sound. This practice energizes the mind as it increases circulation in the brain and gives us the feeling of a "skull shining." It also has a cleansing effect on the breathing pathways and creates heat in the body to stimulate the digestive fire (agni*)*.

Finding Stillness in Silence

You can be in a quiet, peaceful environment without moving your body, yet that does not mean you will find an inner stillness. At times, you will find the opposite, for as soon as you are no longer distracted by your external environment, all of the streams of thought, old stories, and impressions that are currently in your space of mind move into your awareness. Because of this, you may avoid silence through meaningless conversation or seeking constant external stimulation of the senses. When your focus and senses are continuously being stimulated by your environment, you are not able to connect inward. While this can be an unfortunate consequence of not finding quiet moments in your life, it can also be used as an unconscious coping mechanism to avoid having to "deal with" or witness the clutter that has built up in mind space. Yet the effects of a busy mind will ripple out into your energetic and physical body whether you witness them or not, and you will still experience negative outcomes. Avoidance does not remedy a chaotic state of mind.

In silence, we can experience the disengagement of the senses and tune in to our current state of mind. This is the power of silence, the ability to witness the underlying mental activity as it rises to the surface of the conscious mind so we can ungrasp and clear up unnecessary clutter and distractions that cloud mind space. While a quiet, peaceful environment is helpful in reducing distractions, the practice of abiding in silence is not necessarily a space void of noise or sensory deprivation. It is when we are silent, releasing any need to think or respond, that we are at our deepest level of being. We can experience this in our practice, when we are not being led or guided, and sink into being through our personal yoga tools and techniques. It can take place in an immersive experience, such as a retreat, or in simple moments when we are able to just be silent. This is where we can find a deep sense of serenity and tranquility. Our inner stillness is not an empty void of nothingness; it is a balanced unity of everything. Erich Schiffmann reminds us that, "Stillness is dynamic. It is unconflicted movement, life in harmony with itself, skill in action. It can be experienced whenever there is total, uninhibited, unconflicted participation in the moment you are in—when you are wholeheartedly present with whatever you are doing."[31]

Once we are able to find comfort and ease in the silence of our practice, we begin to use the limbs of yoga not only to move through the subtle bodies of the koshas but also to "check in" and connect to each layer. This becomes available through a gradual settling of all of the systems of our living being as we find, connect to, and then abide in our truest form. It is the place where true joy resides and where clarity and deep knowing is found. While the outward draw of the five senses is strong and can cause us to forget our sense of inward perception, our practice reminds us to tune in. Through nurturing our inner stillness, we continue to cultivate clarity and balance throughout our entire being and life. Enjoy the journey!

Afterword

There have been many times in my life when I have felt a shifting occur. Sometimes it has been dramatic and in an instant. For example, I remember after one of my first weekends studying with Michael Stone feeling that it had not *changed* my understanding of practice so much as shifted my entire perspective of practice— what it was, how I could experience it, and how I could share it. It was a clear mental shift…an awakening, perhaps. Then, other times, a shift *needed* to occur and I would fight or resist. For many years, this revealed itself as fear and anxiety within me. My practice was my refuge and my teacher.

Throughout the years, as I furthered my study to learn more to share with my students, it also led to a deep discovery of myself and the world. Practice helped me to witness the opportunities for positive shifts—ways of shedding old stuff and allowing my perspective to widen—and, most importantly, to learn how to be *available to them*. Once I began to experience this freeing release of my grasp on the clouded view of my life through the what-ifs and unknowns, there was the peace that I had longed for. This created another type of shift, an opportunity for change, yet this time it began with a spark of insight and vision. I wanted to share *this* aspect of practice! I felt it loud and clear, and instead of an accompanying feeling of fear, I felt excited.

Guided by this inner spark, I began to envision a space for sharing meditation and the broader view of what yoga encompassed, a space that felt peaceful, calm, and inviting to anyone who entered. I would continue to guide students through poses and breathwork but in a way that was more accessible and purposeful, serving as a tool to move with more ease and depth into meditation. Instead of using just a couple of aspects of practice, I would teach students how to use all of the tools in their specific intended way to obtain all of their benefits, and I would expand my base from those already practicing asana to any "body" who would like help finding ease and balance in their mind. I contemplated the difference in feeling between the environments and energetic qualities of the spaces I visited for meditation retreats compared to the spaces available in my community for practice and came to a realization. I wanted to be able to share the knowledge and experience of how to meditate and find a sense of peace within a *local* retreat space—*a community center for meditation and well-being.*

And so this community center was born and simply named The Meditation Room, with a grounded purpose of sharing the practice and growing my own understanding of how to connect with anyone who was interested—people of all ages, backgrounds, physical abilities, and mental states, from beginning to advanced meditators. My goal was learning how to share meditation with anyone who had a *mind*, so I strived to determine how I could reach, connect with, and teach all. It was a local *retreat-like* environment where the community gathered, learned, and practiced. Throughout this time, I began to dive deeper into how to share the practices of meditation with this broader base. I developed series classes to not only guide students through the experience of meditation but also teach them how to cultivate a personal practice in order to continue growing and expanding its application in their lives. In addition, I designed a teacher training program to help students learn how to share these transformative methods of practice with others. This decade of developing ideas and turning them into a tangible reality at The Meditation Room was a process of experiencing, learning, growing, and shifting. It was a vibrant time of creativity, releasing all that did not serve me and bringing dreams to fruition.

There came a time when I felt another shift occurring, one

that, at first, felt of fatigue and boredom—a curious start, I will admit, to what would be one of my largest creative projects. While this obstacle stemmed from a variety of sources, a shift in how I took care of myself, moved throughout my day, and utilized my creativity and purpose was occurring. I began to look at all that I was teaching, practicing, and learning as a whole. I had tried to write many times in my life before, but it felt forced and would fizzle out before I got too far. This time was different; it just flowed; it felt easeful and enjoyable. Through writing, I knew I could share these life-shifting practices with even more people. My goal has been to guide you through the entire journey of practice, starting at the beginning and leaving you with a sustainable practice for lifelong growth. I hope the teachings of yoga that I have shared, through the lineages of teachers before me, in the pages of this book help you witness and glide through the shifts and opportunities in your life with clarity, calm, and ease.

Om peace,
Jessica

Appendix

Designing a Practice

Step 1: Find a peaceful environment with minimal distractions, if available. Include a mindful ritual such as laying down a blanket and cushion or lighting a candle, sage, palo santo, or incense.

Step 2: Explore a short reading, lesson, or study of a yama, niyama, or sutra. This step can also take place at the end of practice.

Step 3: Find a comfortable meditation seat (that you will return to).

Step 4: Begin to turn your gaze inward to current sensations of body and natural breath.

Step 5: Gradually deepen and lengthen the breath, adding in ocean breath if desired, which you will continue to use through your asana practice.

Step 6: Asana ~ Add gentle movements and postures to your deep, full breath or ocean breath. Make mindful movements of the spine in all directions, then return to your starting meditation seat.

Step 7: Pranayama ~ From your comfortable seat in a still, stable upright position, utilize a specific pranayama technique.

Step 8: Pratyahara ~ Continue to draw your awareness inward and disengage your senses from the distractions of your environment through releasing physical aspects of mental tension.

Step 9: Dharana ~ Allow your mind's eye to rest on an object of attention. Once you notice that your focus has wandered toward a distraction, release your mental grasp and return to the object of attention.

Step 10: Dhyana ~ When there are no longer distractions tugging at your focus, you can gently release your one-pointed focus and sink into a meditative state. If you notice your attention wandering, gently bring your focus to your object of attention to guide you back to this state.

Step 11: Samadhi ~ Abide with ease in your meditative state as your focus and your object of meditation begin to absorb into each other.

Step 12: Living Yoga ~ Experience life from a more easeful and balanced state.

Personalized Practice Plan:

~ Short reading, lesson, or study (at the beginning and/or end of practice)

~ Begin to turn your gaze inward to current sensations of body and natural breath.

- Gradually deepen and lengthen breath (ujjayi pranayama optional).

Asana _____
_____
_____
_____
_____
_____
_____
_____
_____

Pranayama _____

Pratyahara _____

Dharana _____

Dhyana ~ *Merging into oneness with the object of attention.*

Samadhi ~ *Sinking into being and oneness with all that is.*

Sanskrit Glossary

Abhinivesha - the source fear

Agni - fire; digestive fire; transformative power of nature

Ahamkara - ego; sense of identity; the "I"-ness in the mind

Ahimsa - non-violence; a subcategory of the yamas

Anandamaya - bliss sheath; last layer of the koshas that reflects the true Self

Annamaya - body layer; that which is nourished by food; first layer of the koshas

Antarayas - obstacles that arise on the path of yoga

Apana - energetic rubbish that collects when prana is not in a state of equilibrium

Apana-vayu - energetic forces that move away, down, and out

Aparigraha - non-possessiveness; a subcategory of the yamas

Asana - to sit; to establish posture; third limb of yoga practice

Asmita - egoism; "I-am-ness"

Asteya - non-stealing; a subcategory of the yamas

Atman - that which is witnessing; innermost self; soul; the seer and observer of the mind and body

Avidya - ignorance; absence of wisdom

Bhedana - piercing; penetrating

Bhramari - humming (bee) breath

Brahmacharya - non-indulgence; a subcategory of the yamas

Buddhi - aspect of our intellect and wisdom; the ability of the mind to understand, decide, determine, and learn

Chandra - moon

Chitta - consciousness; totality of mind space

Dharana - one-pointed focus; binding our stream of focus to a singular object; sixth limb of yoga practice

Dhyana - meditation; meditative state; seventh limb of yoga practice

Duhkha - bad space; suffering

Dvesha - repulsion; distaste

Gunas - energetic forces; qualities of nature

Hatha Yoga - willful; forceful; the yoga of activity; forceful action to balance sun and moon energies within the body

Ishvara Pranidhana - self-surrender; surrender to divine energy; a subcategory of the niyamas; third foundational element of kriya

Kapalabhati - skull shining breath

Klesha - affliction; poison

Koshas - sheaths or layers of being covering self

Kriya - yoga of action purifying body, energy, and mind

Mana - our ability to take in information through the senses

Manomaya - layer of the automatic mind; nourished by the senses; second layer of the
koshas

Mantra - repetition of a statement; word repeated to aid concentration in meditation (often in Sanskrit)

Mudra - a symbolic hand gesture or pose for an energetic connection

Nadis - channel; flow; network of channels in the body through which energy flows

Namaste - Gesture and phrase translated as, "The light in me honors the light in you."

Niyamas - internal discipline, rules, guidance, or observances; inner self-care; second limb of yoga practice

Prakriti - all that exists in nature; all that has been seen or witnessed; always changing

Prana - life force; a universal energy that flows in currents through living beings

Pranamaya - layer consisting of prana; energetic aspect that animates and brings us to life; second layer of the koshas

Prana-vayu - energetic forces that move forward, inward, and upward

Pranayama - to adjust, shift, and change the prana within; fourth limb of yoga practice

Pratyahara - withdrawal of the senses; gaining control of the senses; fifth limb of yoga practice

Purusha - pure consciousness; true Self; the seer of experience; unchanging

Raga - attachment; desire

Raja Yoga - path toward meditation; eight limbs of yoga practice

Rajas - the quality of activity, passion, and movement; one of the gunas

Sadhana - a daily spiritual practice for achieving a goal

Samadhi - a state of union and oneness with all; eighth limb of yoga practice

Samana-vayu - energetic forces that move from the outside inward

Samskaras - mental impressions

Sanskrit - an ancient language used in spiritual yoga text (such as the *Yoga Sutras*)

Santosha - contentment; deep, lasting fulfillment; subcategory of the niyamas

Sattva - the quality of pure harmony, and balance; one of the gunas

Satya - truthfulness; a subcategory of the yamas

Saucha - purification and cleanliness; a subcategory of the niyamas

Shodhana - cleansing

Sitali - cooling breath

Sthira - the quality of steadiness, strength, and stability

Sukha - good space; happiness, ease, joy, or bliss

Surya - sun

Sutras - string, thread, line, or verse

Svadhyaya - to remember or contemplate oneself; self-study; a subcategory of the niyamas; second foundational element of kriya

Tamas - the quality of dullness, darkness, and inertia; one of the gunas

Tapas - to create or to burn; self-discipline; a subcategory of the niyamas; first foundational element of kriya

Udana-vayu - energetic forces that move out from the heart and upward

Ujjayi Pranayama - victorious breath

Vayus -energetic forces that move in a specific direction and affect different body systems

Vijnanamaya - wisdom sheath; layer of the intellect; nourished by intellect; third layer of the koshas

Villoma - against the natural flow; interrupting the flow of breath

Vyana-vayu - energetic forces that move from the center of the body outward

Yamas - restraint or reining in; self-control or behaviors we refrain from doing; ethical principles; first limb of yoga practice

Yoga - to unite, to yoke, to come together

Notes

Introduction

1. T.K.V. Desikachar, *The Heart of Yoga: Developing a Personal Practice* (Inner Traditions International, 1995), 5.

2. Erich Schiffman, *Yoga: The Spirit and Practice of Moving Into Stillness* (Pocket Books, 1996), 305-6.

Chapter 1: Begin Where You Are

1. Michael Stone, "Looking Within: An Online Meditation Course," 2016, https://michaelstoneteaching.com.

2. Stone, "Looking Within."

Chapter 2: The Practice

1. Desikachar, *Heart of Yoga*, 18.

2. Desikachar, *Heart of Yoga*, 18.

3. Schiffman, "Moving Into Stillness," 47.

4. Desikachar, *Heart of Yoga*, 61.

5. Desikachar, *Heart of Yoga*, 107.

6. Desikachar, *Heart of Yoga*, 109.

7. Desikachar, *Heart of Yoga*, 109.

8. Desikachar, *Heart of Yoga*, 240.

9. Desikachar, *Heart of Yoga*, 240.

10. Desikachar, *Heart of Yoga*, 110.

Chapter 3: The Journey

1. Michael Stone, *The Inner Tradition of Yoga: A Guide to Yoga Philosophy for the Contemporary Practitioner* (Shambhala Publications, 2018), 99-100.

2. Stone, "Inner Tradition," 99-100.

3. Vasant Dattatray Lad, Fundamental Principles of Ayurveda, vol.1 of Textbook of Ayurveda (The Ayurvedic Press, 2002), 194.

4. Lad, Principles Ayurveda, 1:194.

5. Lad, Principles Ayurveda, 1:194.

6. Lad, Principles Ayurveda, 1:195.

7. Lad, Principles Ayurveda, 1:195.

8. Danny Penman, "Can Mindfulness Meditation Really Reduce Pain and Suffering?", *Psychology Today*, January 9, 2015, https://www.psychologytoday.com/us/blog/mindfulness-in-frantic-world/201501/can-mindfulness-meditation-really-reduce-pain-and-suffering.

9. Swami Jnaneshvara Bharati, "Yoga Sutras 2.54-2.55: Pratyahara of Sense Withdrawal, Rung #5 of 8," Swami J, September 5, 2025, https://swamij.com/yoga-sutras-25455.htm#2.54.

Chapter 4: Deepening the Connection

1. Erich Schiffman, conversation with author in Yogaville class in Buckingham, Virginia, 2016.

2. Desikachar, *Heart of Yoga*, 97.

3. Desikachar, *Heart of Yoga*, 98.

4. Desikachar, *Heart of Yoga*, 98.

5. Ram Dass and Stephen Levine, *Grist for the Mill* (Unity Press, 1977), ix.

6. Desikachar, *Heart of Yoga*, 99.

7. Desikachar, *Heart of Yoga*, 99.

8. Desikachar, *Heart of Yoga*, 99.

9. Desikachar, *Heart of Yoga*, 100.

10. Desikachar, *Heart of Yoga*, 97.

11. Timothy Burgin, "The Five Niyamas of Yoga: Definition & Practice Tips," *Yoga Basics*, October 13, 2020, https://www.yogabasics.com/learn/the-five-niyamas-of-yoga/.

12. Stone, "Inner Tradition," 46.

13. Desikachar, *Heart of Yoga*, 101.

14. Desikachar, *Heart of Yoga*, 101.

15. Desikachar, *Heart of Yoga*, 101.

16. Desikachar, *Heart of Yoga*, 101.

17. Desikachar, *Heart of Yoga*, 101.

18. Desikachar, *Heart of Yoga*, 101-2.

19. Desikachar, *Heart of Yoga*, 17.

20. Desikachar, *Heart of Yoga*, 109.

21. Michael Stone, *Awake in the World: Teachings from Yoga and Buddhism for Living an Engaged Life* (Shambhala Publications, 2011), 4.

Chapter 5: Intertwining of Our Being

1. Stone, "Inner Tradition," 127.

2. Stone, "Inner Tradition," 127.

3. Desikachar, *Heart of Yoga*, 57.

4. Desikachar, *Heart of Yoga*, 57.

5. Lad, Principles Ayurveda, 1:15.

6. Stone, "Inner Tradition," 151.

7. Lad, Principles Ayurveda, 1:197.

8. Lad, Principles Ayurveda, 1:8.

9. Stone, "Inner Tradition," 151.

10. Stone, "Inner Tradition," 130.

11. Paramhansa Atmananda, "Chitta Suddhi (Inner Purification)," *From Guruji's Desk* (blog), *Kriya Yoga Jagat*, October 24, 2018. https://kriyayogajagat.com/chitta-suddhi/.

Chapter 6: Calming the Fluctuations of Mind

1. Desikachar, *Heart of Yoga*, 149. Translation of sutra 1.1 of the *Yoga Sutras of Patanjali*: "Here begins the authoritative instruction on Yoga."

2. Desikachar, *Heart of Yoga*, 149. Translation of sutra 1.2 of the *Yoga Sutras of Patanjali*: "Yoga is the ability to direct the mind exclusively toward an object and sustain that direction without any distractions."

3. Desikachar, *Heart of Yoga*, 150. Translation of sutra 1.3 of the *Yoga Sutras of Patanjali*: "Then the ability to understand the object fully and correctly is apparent."

4. Desikachar, *Heart of Yoga*, 150. Translation of sutra 1.4 of the *Yoga Sutras of Patanjali*: "The ability to understand the object is simply replaced by the mind's conception of that object or by a total lack of comprehension."

5. Desikachar, *Heart of Yoga*, 153. Translation of sutra 1.12 of the *Yoga Sutras of Patanjali*: "The mind can reach the state of Yoga through practice and detachment."

6. Desikachar, *Heart of Yoga*, 153. Translation of sutra 1.12 of the *Yoga Sutras of Patanjali*: "The mind can reach the state of Yoga through practice and detachment."

7. Desikachar, *Heart of Yoga*, 121.

8. Desikachar, *Heart of Yoga*, 121.

9. Desikachar, *Heart of Yoga*, 121.

10. Desikachar, *Heart of Yoga*, 121.

11. Desikachar, *Heart of Yoga*, 122.

12. Stone, "Inner Tradition," 226.

13. Huruki Murakami, *What I Talk About When I Talk About Running* (Knopf Doubleday Publishing Group, 2009), 82.

14. Desikachar, *Heart of Yoga*, 80.

15. Desikachar, *Heart of Yoga*, 80.

16. Desikachar, *Heart of Yoga*, 80.

17. Desikachar, *Heart of Yoga*, 80.

18. Desikachar, *Heart of Yoga*, 80.

19. Desikachar, *Heart of Yoga*, 165. Translation of sutra 2.2 of the *Yoga Sutras of Patanjali*: "Then such practices will be certain to remove obstacles to clear perception."

20. Stone, "Inner Tradition," 228.

21. Desikachar, *Heart of Yoga*, 161. Translation of sutra 1.41 of the *Yoga Sutras of Patanjali*: "When the mind is free from distraction, it is possible for all the mental processes to be involved in the object of inquiry."

22. Desikachar, *Heart of Yoga*, 17.

23. Stone, "Inner Tradition," 83.

24. Desikachar, *Heart of Yoga*, 163. Translation of sutra 1.47 of the *Yoga Sutras of Patanjali*: "Then the individual begins to truly know himself."

Chapter 7: Guidebook to Caring for Self

1. Desikachar, *Heart of Yoga*, 123.

2. Desikachar, *Heart of Yoga*, 85.

3. Desikachar, *Heart of Yoga*, 93.

4. Rolf Sovik, "The Gunas: Nature's Three Fundamental Forces," Yoga International, October 1, 2025, https://yogainternational.com/article/view/the-gunas-natures-three-fundamental-forces/.

5. Desikachar, *Heart of Yoga*, 85.

6. Desikachar, *Heart of Yoga*, 85.

7. Desikachar, *Heart of Yoga*, 125.

8. B.K.S. Iyengar, *Light on Life: The Yoga Journey to Wholeness, Inner Peace, and Ultimate Freedom* (Rodale Books, 2005), 167.

9. Desikachar, *Heart of Yoga*, 14.

10. Desikachar, *Heart of Yoga*, 80.

11. Desikachar, *Heart of Yoga*, 58.

12. Desikachar, *Heart of Yoga*, 62.

13. Desikachar, *Heart of Yoga*, 165. Translation from the *Yoga Sutras of Patanjali* of sutras 2.2 (see note 19 from Chapter 6) and 2.1: "The practice of Yoga must reduce both

physical and mental impurities. It must develop our capacity for self-examination and help us to understand that, in the final analysis, we are not the masters of everything we do."

14. Desikachar, *Heart of Yoga*, 80.

15. Desikachar, *Heart of Yoga*, 165. Translation of sutras 2.1-2.2 of the *Yoga Sutras of Patanjali*.

16. Desikachar, *Heart of Yoga*, 165. Translation of sutras 2.1-2.2 of the *Yoga Sutras of Patanjali*.

17. Desikachar, *Heart of Yoga*, 13.

18. Desikachar, *Heart of Yoga*, 165. Translation of sutras 2.1-2.2 of the *Yoga Sutras of Patanjali*.

19. Desikachar, *Heart of Yoga*, 165. Translation of sutras 2.1-2.2 of the *Yoga Sutras of Patanjali*.

20. Desikachar, *Heart of Yoga*, 137.

21. Kevin Parenteau, "Yin Yoga Explained: A Guide to the History, Practice, and Benefits," *Beginner Yoga Blog, Asana at Home Online Yoga*, December 5, 2023. https://asanaathome.com/yin-yoga-explained/.

22. Judith Hanson Lasater, *Relax and Renew: Restful Yoga for Stressful Times* (Rodmell Press, 1995), 6.

23. Desikachar, *Heart of Yoga*, 57.

24. Desikachar, *Heart of Yoga*, 58.

25. Timothy Burgin, "Surya Bhedana Pranayama: Sun-Piercing Breath," *Yoga Basics*, January 5, 2024, https://www.yogabasics.com/practice/pranayama/surya-bhedana-pranayama/.

26. Timothy Burgin, "Chandra Bhedana Pranayama: Moon-Piercing Breath," *Yoga Basics*, January 2, 2024, https://www.yogabasics.com/practice/pranayama/chandra-bhedana-pranayama/.

27. Desikachar, *Heart of Yoga*, 61.

28. Prana Editors, "Viloma Pranayama in Yoga," Prana Sutra, April 24, 2025, https://www.prana-sutra.com/post/viloma-pranayama-interrupted-breathing.

29. Prana Editors, "Bhramari Pranayama Benefits and How to Do the Humming Bee Breath in Yoga," Prana Sutra, October 22, 2025, https://www.prana-sutra.com/post/bhramari-pranayama-steps-benefits.

30. Desikachar, *Heart of Yoga*, 62.

31. Schiffman, "Moving Into Stillness," 3.

Bibliography

Atmananda, Paramhansa. 2018. "Chitta Suddhi (Inner Purification)." *From Guruji's Desk* (blog), October 24, 2018. https://kriyayogajagat.com/chitta-suddhi/.

Bacci, Ingrid. *The Art of Effortless Living*. Tarcher, 2002.

Bharati, Swami Jnaneshvara. "Yoga Sutras 2.54-2.55: Pratyahara of Sense Withdrawal, Rung #5 of 8." Accessed September 5, 2025. https://swamij.com/yoga-sutras-25455.htm#2.54.

Burgin, Timothy. "The Five Niyamas of Yoga: Definition & Practice Tips." Yoga Basics. Published on October 13, 2020. https://www.yogabasics.com/learn/the-five-niyamas-of-yoga/.

Burgin, Timothy. "Chandra Bhedana Pranayama: Moon-Piercing Breath." Yoga Basics. Published on January 2, 2024. https://www.yogabasics.com/practice/pranayama/chandra-bhedana-pranayama/.

Burgin, Timothy. "Surya Bhedana Pranayama: Sun-Piercing Breath." Yoga Basics. Published on January 5, 2024. https://www.yogabasics.com/practice/pranayama/surya-bhedana-pranayama/.

Dass, Ram, and Stephen Levine. *Grist for the Mill*. Unity Press, 1977.

Desikachar, T.K.V. *The Heart of Yoga: Developing a Personal Practice.* Inner Traditions International, 1995.

Iyengar, B.K.S. *Light on Life: The Yoga Journey to Wholeness, Inner Peace, and Ultimate Freedom.* Rodale Books, 2005.

Lad, Vasant Dattatray. *Fundamental Principles of Ayurveda.* Vol.1 of *Textbook of Ayurveda.* The Ayurvedic Press, 2002.

Lasater, Judith Hanson. *Relax and Renew: Restful Yoga for Stressful Times.* Rodmell Press, 1995.

Murakami, Huruki. *What I Talk About When I Talk About Running.* Knopf Doubleday Publishing Group, 2009.

Parenteau, Kevin. 2023. "Yin Yoga Explained: A Guide to the History, Practice, and Benefits." *Beginner Yoga Blog*, December 5, 2023. https://asanaathome.com/yin-yoga-explained/.

Penman, Danny. 2015. "Can Mindfulness Meditation Really Reduce Pain and Suffering?" *Psychology Today*, January 9. https://www.psychologytoday.com/us/blog/mindfulness-in-frantic-world/201501/can-mindfulness-meditation-really-reduce-pain-and-suffering.

Prana Editors. "Viloma Pranayama in Yoga." Prana Sutra, Updated April 24, 2025. https://www.prana-sutra.com/post/viloma-pranayama-interrupted-breathing.

Prana Editors. "Bhramari Pranayama Benefits and How to Do the Humming Bee Breath in Yoga." Prana Sutra,

Accessed October 22, 2025. https://www.prana-
sutra.com/post/bhramari-pranayama-steps-benefits.

Schiffmann, Erich. *Yoga: The Spirit and Practice of Moving Into
Stillness*. Pocket Books, 1996.

Sovik, Rolf. "The Gunas: Nature's Three Fundamental
Forces." Yoga International, Accessed October 1, 2025.
https://yogainternational.com/article/view/the-gunas-
natures-three-fundamental-forces/.

Stone, Michael. *Awake in the World: Teachings from Yoga and
Buddhism for Living an Engaged Life*. Shambhala
Publications, 2011.

Stone, Michael. "Looking Within: An Online Meditation Course."
Accessed 2016, https://michaelstoneteaching.com.

Stone, Michael. *The Inner Tradition of Yoga: A Guide to Yoga
Philosophy for the Contemporary Practitioner*. Shambhala
Publications, 2018.

About the Author

Jessica Bowles began her personal yoga practice in 1996, as a teenager living in the suburbs of West Virginia, through the study of Erich Schiffmann's book *Yoga: The Spirit and Practice of Moving Into Stillness* and the video *Yoga Mind & Body* with Ali MacGraw. She is forever grateful that, in a time when yoga was emerging into communities through asana, he presented and shared the foundation of yoga's true purpose of uniting with self through meditation. In 2006, after moving to Charlotte, North Carolina, Jessica discovered a local teacher training led by Lesa Crocker, who had been trained by Erich. Jessica completed her 230-Hour Registered Yoga Teacher credential through Bodhi Tree Yoga School and began the journey of teaching weekly classes while continuing her education, later receiving her 500-Hour RYT credential from Asheville Yoga Center. It was at this time that she met Michael Stone, who led the weekend on the *Yoga Sutras*. His teachings on the depth of practice prompted an immense shift in Jessica's personal understanding of yoga and expanded the ways in which she could share meditation with others.

In 2009, Jessica studied Thai Yoga Therapy with Saul David Raye at Ritam Healing Arts in Ojai, California, and experienced the capacity of the body and mind to heal and rejuvenate. She then received her 625-Hour Ayurveda Wellness Counselor credential from Kerala Ayurveda Academy in 2010, which allowed her to understand the depths of how our daily routines and habits create our current state of being. She also traveled annually to study with Michael Stone up until his sudden passing in 2017 as well as with Erich Schiffmann before his teaching hiatus that same year. This was a time of immense shedding of old ideas and habits while, at the same time, learning through a clearer, expanding view.

In 2015, Jessica opened The Meditation Room in hopes of creating a center for meditation in her local community of Lake

Norman, North Carolina. Today, Jessica continues to share with others the ability to heal and change self-destructive patterns of the mind and clear the mental clutter that accumulates by practicing meditation and yoga. Her passion and practice shine through as she shares techniques, practices, and the wisdom of yoga philosophy through tangible teachings that relate to modern-day living and can be easily infused into everyday life.

www.ingramcontent.com/pod-product-compliance
Lightning Source LLC
Chambersburg PA
CBHW020202090426
42734CB00008B/914